NATIONAL INSTITUTE SOCIAL SERVICES LIBRARY

Volume 5

COMMUNITY WORK

COMMUNITY WORK
Learning and Supervision

Edited by
CATHERINE BRISCOE AND
DAVID N. THOMAS

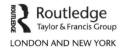

Routledge
Taylor & Francis Group

LONDON AND NEW YORK

First published in 1977 by George Allen & Unwin Ltd

This edition first published in 2022
by Routledge
4 Park Square, Milton Park, Abingdon, Oxon OX14 4RN
605 Third Avenue, New York, NY 10017

Routledge is an imprint of the Taylor & Francis Group, an informa business

© 1977 by Taylor & Francis.

British Library Cataloguing in Publication Data
A catalogue record for this book is available from the British Library

ISBN: 978-1-03-203381-5 (Set)
ISBN: 978-1-00-321681-0 (Set) (ebk)
ISBN: 978-1-03-204175-9 (Volume 5) (hbk)
ISBN: 978-1-03-204190-2 (Volume 5) (pbk)
ISBN: 978-1-00-319084-4 (Volume 5) (ebk)

DOI: 10.4324/9781003190844

Publisher's Note
The publisher has gone to great lengths to ensure the quality of this reprint but points out that some imperfections in the original copies may be apparent.

Disclaimer
The publisher has made every effort to trace copyright holders and would welcome correspondence from those they have been unable to trace.

COMMUNITY WORK: LEARNING AND SUPERVISION

Edited by

CATHERINE BRISCOE

Visiting Senior Lecturer in Social Work,
University of Singapore

and

DAVID N. THOMAS

Lecturer in Community Work,
National Institute for Social Work

London
GEORGE ALLEN & UNWIN LTD
RUSKIN HOUSE   MUSEUM STREET

First published in 1977

ISBN 0 04 361026 9 (Hardback)
0 04 361027 7 (Paperback)

Printed in Great Britain
in 10 on 11 pt Times Roman
by
Willmer Brothers Limited, Birkenhead

Skill comes so slow and life so fast doth fly
We learn so little and forget so much

Sir John Davis
Nosce Teipsum, Introduction XIX

ACKNOWLEDGEMENTS

We are grateful to Peter Righton, David Jones, David Cooke and Elizabeth Thomas for reading and commenting on papers; to Diana Broad, Priscilla Foley, Jenny McElhinney, Rosina Shaw, Margaret Theodore, Ruby Woodman and secretarial staff at the National Institute for Social Work for help in typing and preparing the papers; to Maureen Webley for tracking down references and relevant material; to our colleagues for their time in discussing the book and supporting our endeavours; to our former course members at the National Institute whose perspectives on, and reactions to, the training for which we were responsible provided the initiative for this book; and, most of all, to those who provided the papers, with special thanks for their patience in accepting our editorial suggestions and idiosyncrasies.

CONTENTS

NOTES ON CONTRIBUTORS

JIMMY ALGIE is Senior Lecturer in Management and Organisation Studies at the National Institute for Social Work.

PETER BALDOCK is Principal Social Worker (Community Development) in the Family and Community Services Department, Sheffield.

CATHERINE BRISCOE is Senior Lecturer in Social Work Methods at the University of Singapore. She was previously a Lecturer in Community Work at the National Institute for Social Work.

RICHARD BRYANT is a Fieldwork Teacher at the Crossroads Youth and Community Association, Glasgow.

NICHOLAS DERRICOURT is Senior Lecturer in Community Work at Sunderland Polytechnic. He was previously a Senior Lecturer in Community Work at the City of Birmingham Polytechnic.

JALNA HANMER is Lecturer in Community Work at the London School of Economics and Political Science.

PATRICK HARRIS is Community Work Co-ordinator in the London Borough of Hackney.

BARBARA HOLMES is a Fieldwork Teacher at the Crossroads Youth and Community Association, Glasgow.

NORMAN KAM is Professional Adviser to the Director of Social Welfare, Hong Kong.

JOHN LAMBERT is a Lecturer in the Department of Social Administration, University College, Cardiff. He was previously Senior Lecturer in Sociology at the City of Birmingham Polytechnic.

PETER LEONARD is Professor of Applied Social Studies in the University of Warwick.

NANO McCAUGHAN is Lecturer in Social Group Work at the National Institute for Social Work.

CLIVE MILLER is Lecturer in Management and Organisation Studies at the National Institute for Social Work.

HARRY SALMON is Community Work Tutor at the Community Work Centre, Coventry.

DAVID THOMAS is Lecturer in Community Work at the National Institute for Social Work.

WILLIAM WARBURTON is a Research Officer at the National Institute for Social Work.

INTRODUCTION

In the past decade, there has been a rapid development of interest in community work and its practice in a variety of settings. The experience gained from that practice is increasingly being described, defined and debated. The Gulbenkian Group has provided broad overviews of the field.[1] The Association of Community Workers has encouraged and published descriptions of particular aspects of practice.[2] Independent and experimental projects publish accounts of the development and process of their work. The Community Development Projects are preparing extensive reports on the context of community work, the problems faced by those with whom community workers are involved and the resistances of those who control resources and decision making.[3] These analyses are used to clarify goals and strategies available to practitioners. Professional journals are also giving generous coverage to aspects of practice, and publications such as *Community Action*[4] and the papers of the National Council of Social Service provide further forums for pooling information and sharing learning from experience.

The steady flow of analyses of practice shows the eagerness of community workers to share with one another, and to develop a wider understanding of, the possibilities and problems of community work. This clarification, however, has begun to highlight the controversial issues in the field as well as some areas of general agreement.

TRAINING ISSUES

One question which arouses fierce emotions is the training and personal qualifications of those who practise community work. The Central Council for Education and Training in Social Work[5] and the Association of Community Workers[6] have recently published detailed accounts of the knowledge and skills that are required by community workers in order for them to be effective in their job and of use to those with whom they work. These descriptions were developed by different groups of experienced community work practitioners and trainers who had come to recognise the complexity of community work tasks and the personal resources necessary for the practitioner who undertakes them.

These papers have aroused heated reactions[7] from some practitioners who express fear and rejection of the 'professionalisation' of community work. The fears relate to:

the distancing power of theory. It is feared that the worker who acquires too much theory about social problems and human behaviour may stand outside situations and analyse them as an observer rather than feel himself to be in the situation and committed to changing it. It is thought that academic theories describe and explain phenomena without giving any help as to how to change them. It is also felt that understanding could give power to manipulate those with whom the community worker works and who are directly involved in and affected by the situation;

the exclusivity of training. It is argued that emphasis on the need for knowledge and skills perpetuates training courses offering qualifications in community work, and situated in higher education institutions which usually demand prequalifications of O and A levels and sometimes a degree or previous professional qualification. Such courses exclude many people, particularly those from deprived areas where education is one of the many inadequate resources. It is feared that such courses may make community work just one more white-collar job for those coming from comfortable and well provided backgrounds and exclude those whom community work is supposedly most concerned to help;

the upward mobility of the trained. It is suggested that the qualified community worker may use 'the community' as a stepping stone to a highly paid administrative or educational post where he will be an expert in the needs of the disadvantaged. In a local authority department or field organisation his or her salary may be drawn from funds allocated for meeting needs. Power holders and decision makers may turn to him for information on the needs of the disadvantaged rather than consulting them direct.

These fears partly represent the British community worker's pre-occupation[8] with preserving community work as an ideologically based social movement which requires emotional commitment rather than planning and structure and partly express concerns which are real and are experienced by many practitioners and community residents.

Existing disciplines such as the social and political sciences are only beginning to focus on the needs and perspectives of the disadvantaged. Those who seek knowledge in this area must hunt through much irrelevant material to find useful and applicable learning. The exclusivity of present patterns of education, and the process by which the successful jumping of a series of exam hurdles offers qualifications which give entry to professional career structures, do restrict and constrain the employment and social mobility of community residents. Not only community work but other occupational areas of equal or greater importance are effectively closed to them as a result of the present distribution of educational resources.

However, it is a simplistic response to this situation to deny that community workers need to have any resources of knowledge and skills or access to training opportunities whereby these resources can be developed and improved. It belittles the reality of the problems confronting those with whom community workers work. Those practitioners and trainers who recognise community work as a series of complex tasks, which demand knowledge and skill for their effective performance, see clearly the scope of the problems with which community residents are faced and the difficulty of finding feasible strategies to cope with them. But these practitioners and trainers are also struggling to define:

1 the parts of known theory that are useful to the practice of community work;
2 how those particular areas of knowledge can best be communicated to all those engaged in community work tasks. This is a difficult undertaking because community workers who wish to develop for themselves and to share with community residents the understanding derived from established bodies of knowledge will have to wrestle with concepts and models often shrouded in obscure language. The response of the community worker to this difficulty can be either to reject knowledge and knowledge seeking or to work at developing means of communication which will help both practitioners and community residents acquire and use knowledge to facilitate the achievement of their goals;
3 the training processes that help in the integration of knowledge with practice and in the development of community work skills. Given the fears and resistances described above, this too is a question fraught with problems.

The CCETSW and ACW papers are contributions to this struggle. They provide a general response to the first question on the knowledge and skills useful to community work. The ACW paper also touches on the issue of specifying and adapting particular areas of knowledge.

The last two questions are presently being explored. The ACW, various practitioners' groups and voluntary organisations are considering apprenticeship schemes for prospective community workers as a training pattern which would help in the integration of knowledge and practice. Community workers in the field are exploring with their employers and with teachers from various institutions the ways in which they can have access to new knowledge and can develop their practice skills.

THIS BOOK

As teachers in an institute which has had a comparatively long involvement in training for community work, we are developing training both for students of community work and for practitioners in the field. We consider the three areas of definition outlined above as vital to the development of community work as a process which can be effective in bringing about social change. We believe training should be a way of raising the level of consciousness of community workers and not of deadening their commitment. To this extent, we believe in dialogical education and training that '. . . strives for the *emergence* of consciousness and *critical intervention* in reality.'[9]

This collection of papers is a contribution to discussion on the knowledge that community workers can use to improve their practice and on the means available to communicate and develop knowledge and skill.

We have asked practitioners and trainers to look at various aspects of theory or at various training processes for developing practice and to consider their contribution to community work.

We have considered in Parts I and III some training processes open to practitioners and to students. In Part I we have concentrated on the practitioner and have looked at training instruments developed by practitioners and by their employing organisations. These chapters focus on the uses and on the problems of these instruments in improving practice skills and knowledge. In Part III we have focused on the field practice of students. These chapters consider the possibilities and problems of different aspects of field placement. We have not been able in either of these Parts to include anything on simulation gaming, the uses of video for skill training or the development of recording and evaluation methods for community work activities. These have been developed by some practitioners and trainers as useful tools for developing practice skills and we include some references at the end of this introduction.

In Part II we concentrate on areas of knowledge which seem to be particularly susceptible to suspicions that theory can be either irrelevant or dangerously manipulative. Knowledge of politics, planning and social policy is generally accepted as necessary for community work but subjects such as management studies, group theory and research techniques are often seen as tools of power holders to control and quieten demands for change. However, we can find in these subjects concepts and frameworks that help the community worker make sense of the diverse situations in which he is involved and indicate how he can order the complexity of his activity. Management studies offer him insights on organisational behaviour and resistances to change as well as possible frameworks for choice of goals and strategies. Group theory helps him understand the motivations of group members and what keeps them involved in, or pushes them out of, group activity. Research methods can be used to help community groups understand the variety of problems and interests experienced by the residents of their own locality. The chapters on these knowledge areas highlight aspects which seem to have particular relevance to community work and guide the reader to further writings on these subjects.

We hope that practitioners and trainers will find this selection of papers helpful in developing ideas and ways of training that can be used in their own practice development. We want to encourage others to write about their experience of methods of training that have helped them to improve practice, and of theory that has helped them to understand and work in the complex field of community work.

REFERENCES

1 Gulbenkian Group. *Community Work and Social Change* (Longmans 1968); *Current Issues in Community Work* (Routledge & Kegan Paul, 1973).

2 David Jones and Marjorie Mayo (eds), *Community Work One* and *Community Work Two* (Routledge & Kegan Paul, 1974, 1975); Association of Community Workers, *Talking Point*, series of discussion papers circulated at irregular intervals).

3 Community Development Projects, occasional papers from various projects, e.g. Coventry, Newham; and *Inter-Project Report* 1974 (CDP Information and Intelligence Unit, 1974).

4 *Community Action* (an independent bi-monthly journal, P.O. Box 665, London, SW1 8DZ).

5 Central Council for Education and Training in Social Work, *The Teaching of Community Work* (CCETSW Paper 8, 1975).

6 Association of Community Workers, *Knowledge and Skills for Community Work* (ACW, 1975).

7 For example, 'The Professional Goon Show', in *Community Action* No. 24 (August–September 1975).

8 As described by Harry Specht, 'The Dilemma of Community Work in the United Kingdom: A Comment' published in *Policy and Politics* vol. 4 No. 1 (September 1975).

9 Paulo Freire, *Pedagogy of the Oppressed* (Penguin, London, 1973), p. 54.

FURTHER READING

Recording
George W. Goetschius, *Working with Community Groups* (Routledge & Kegan Paul, 1969), pp. 111–29.

Arthur Dunham, *Community Welfare Organizing* (Thos. Y. Crowell Co., New York, 1958), chapter 18.

Roger Mitton and Elizabeth Morrison, *A Community Project in Notting Dale* (Allen Lane Penguin Press, 1972), appendix.

Peter Baldock, *Community Work and Social Work* (Routledge & Kegan Paul, 1974), chapter 6.

Gulbenkian Group, *Current Issues in Community Work* (Routledge & Kegan Paul, 1973), chapter 5.

Use of Video
John Hopkins *et al.*, *Video in Community Development* (Ovum Ltd, London, 1972).
'*Video: Can it Help?*', in *Community Action* No. 22 (June–July 1975).
Inter-Action Advisory Service, *Basic Video in Community Work*, Handbook No. 5 (Inter-Action Imprint, London, 1975).

Simulation Gaming and Laboratory Work
Jack Rothman and Wyatt Jones, *A New Look at Field Instruction* (Association Press, New York, 1971).

PART I

DEVELOPING PRACTICE:
THE WORKER

INTRODUCTION TO PART I

Training and learning do not come to an end at the conclusion of the community worker's period of study. Students will continue to develop their knowledge and skills 'on the job', as community workers employed in an agency or by a community group. Indeed, many community workers do not have any training other than that which they acquire in service, and other professionals working in the community are usually able to develop the community work component of their jobs only through opportunities presented in the course of their work.

Many writers have stressed the value of in-service training,[1] and the chapter by David Thomas and William Warburton outlines the different opportunities for staff development that are available for community workers in social service departments. Many of these opportunities are available in the other settings in which community workers are employed such as planning, housing and chief executive departments, and a variety of voluntary agencies. Thomas and Warburton discuss the use that is made of supervision, consultants and community workers' groups, and in the subsequent papers each of these opportunities for staff development is explored in more detail. Patrick Harris discusses the contribution of agency-based supervision; Catherine Briscoe treats the role and work of the community work consultant; and Peter Baldock reviews the opportunities for training that may be found in community workers' groups. Each of these chapters attempts to analyse the current situation in respect of supervision, consultancy and peer group support, and each presents specific recommendations that are relevant to community workers and those responsible for their ongoing learning and development.

The chapter by Patrick Harris examines the administrative, educative and supportive aspects of the community work supervisor's task. Harris argues that 'a supervisor should strive to help his community workers become more independent, self-critical and self-directing'. The paper indicates that there are many factors which may frustrate this objective, including the supervisor's commitment to his agency and the community worker's political views and loyalty to the community groups with whom he works.

Catherine Briscoe suggests that consultancy is a way of promoting and developing community work practice. She explores the types of help that community work consultants are asked to give. These include planning, training, conflict mediation and confirming values and goals. The chapter also presents a process of consultation that includes a checklist of tasks for the consultant and the community worker. The final chapter in this section is by Peter Baldock. He examines the composition and tasks of community workers' groups. He suggests that very few of the tasks undertaken in community workers' groups relate to professional development or training. Baldock indicates some of the difficulties that these groups encounter in taking on a training function, suggests some solutions and concludes with the view that the role of community workers' groups in training is necessarily limited.

REFERENCE

1 See for instance John Ward, 'In-Service Community Work Training: A Job-Centred Approach', in D. Jones and M. Mayo (eds), *Community Work Two* (Routledge & Kegan Paul, 1975).

Chapter 1

STAFF DEVELOPMENT IN COMMUNITY WORK IN SOCIAL SERVICE DEPARTMENTS*

David N. Thomas and R. William Warburton

An important task in any organisation that delivers goods or services is that of monitoring, and helping to enhance, the quality of the work of its employees. In the social services the motivation for quality control does not come from a possible loss of patronage if standards decline and services deteriorate. Rather, it is largely dependent on the standards individual agencies or departments set themselves and the motivation of individual staff members.

Social services departments attempt to develop the competency of their staff through a variety of mechanisms. These include supervision with the Area Officer or a senior social worker; general discussion opportunities of an informal nature with colleagues; in-service training in the form of attendance at courses and seminars; and the provision of a consultant, often from outside the department. Standards of practice may also be improved by the individual himself through learning from experience, working and observing others and through reading and private study.

In the remainder of this chapter we shall suggest some of the factors that influence both the provision of such opportunities and the use made of them by community workers. It is our contention that many community workers are not, and do not wish to be, influenced by those mechanisms which have traditionally been used in social work agencies to improve the practice of their staff. We suggest, for instance, that supervision and other discussion opportunities are inadequately exploited by community workers and their departments.

THE PROVISION OF OPPORTUNITIES

The scale and quality of the provision of in-service training opportunities will be affected by a number of factors that derive from the nature of the

* This chapter draws upon contacts and discussions with groups of community workers where members are attached to area groups. Many of the ideas that we put forward are being further explored by us, but we feel it might be of use to share them at this early stage.

organisation in which the community worker operates. These will include, but are not limited to:

the culture and tradition in the department in respect of ongoing education and training;
the resources available to the department. For instance, the size of the budget allocated for staff training, as well as the expertise that is available both internally and externally. Many departments and agencies may find it difficult to find people sufficiently experienced in community work for tasks such as staff consultancy;
the department's perception of community work. It is not uncommon to find confusion in the social services about the nature, goals and methods of community work. To the extent that these are unclear, it will be correspondingly difficult to identify and provide for the development of community work staff. In this respect, the presence of a community work adviser at a senior management level may help towards the provision of in-service training opportunities.

THE USE OF DISCUSSION OPPORTUNITIES

In this section we shall look particularly at the use made by community workers of supervision meetings and of informal opportunities to discuss their work with colleagues. We shall refer to both kinds of opportunities for skill development and knowledge promotion as *discussion opportunities*.

The use by community workers of discussion opportunities will largely be determined by *the relationship between a community worker and his social work colleagues*. This relationship will in turn be fashioned by a variety of factors, amongst which we select the following as important for community workers in area groups of social service departments:

1 the office of the community worker within the organisation of the area group. An office 'is a point (location) in organisational space defined by one or more roles (and thereby one or more activities) intended for performance by a single individual. It locates the individual in relation to his fellows with respect to the job to be done and the giving and taking of orders';[1]
2 the training and work background of the community worker;
3 the goals and values of the community worker;
4 the basis of the authority of the community worker's supervisor;
5 the community worker's sources of authority;
6 the role orientation of the community worker.

The office of the community worker
It may be the case that the readiness of a department to provide, and that of community workers to use, discussion opportunities will depend in part

upon the extent to which the community worker is seen, and sees himself, as part of the area group within which he works. It is our view that many community workers in social service departments are only marginal members of their area groups, and that their office is usually located on the boundary of the area group organisation. Many community workers seem to be members of the department only insofar as it pays their salaries, provides minimal resources such as a desk and telephone, and gives some general mandate for their work. We believe that the neighbourhood interventions of many community workers are 'grafted' on to the social services department and that their area group is, in effect, a 'host' system for a range of goals, values, strategies and activities that remain unintegrated within those of the department.[2]

The community worker, unlike his social work colleagues, is relatively free of devices which manage the import of problems upon which he works and which control the quality of the service that he gives. Whereas intake teams or allocation meetings distribute individual cases to particular social workers, the community worker makes decisions himself about the work he will take on. We have found little evidence that these decisions are made with reference to the views of colleagues, or to the overall goals or priorities (where they are articulated) of the area group.

In addition, many community workers are not fully members of a team within their area group; they often describe themselves as 'attached' or 'allocated' to a team, sometimes on a rota basis. Community workers seem in most cases to be directly responsible to the Area Officer and often they have direct access to people further up the hierarchy, like an Assistant Director. Whatever the value of this access to the worker's activities, it certainly serves to heighten his distinctive position in the area group structure.

The boundary office of a community worker in an area group is often a source of anxiety and community workers talk frequently of their feelings of isolation. It also exacerbates worries about conflicting loyalties to department and community groups: many community workers, feeling isolated, vague about their duties and uncertain about their area group's expectations, will expend much time and energy in attacking the department but without recognising it as a resource to aid their decisions and develop skills and knowledge.

The training and background of the community worker
We suggest that a community worker's experience in social work, if any at all, as well as his previous education and training for community work, if any, will help to determine whether or not he will be able to identify with (and be influenced by) the importance given within the social services department to the monitoring and enhancement of the competence of staff. Community workers with some form of social work training and with

some previous experience as caseworkers may be more ready to accept the responsibility of the department, and the contributions of their area group colleagues, to further skill and knowledge. Such workers, through their previous experience of social work, may be in a state of 'role readiness' and thus be more willing to accept the authority of the department, and the opportunities given by working in it, in respect of staff development.[3] In effect, they will have been socialised to the culture of the social services department and be more willing and able to respond positively to those elements of the culture that attach importance to quality control and improvement.

The goals and values of the community worker
It may be hypothesised that the readiness of community workers to make use of discussion opportunities presented within their departments will also be determined by the extent to which the community worker subscribes, if at all, to its significant goals and norms, and perhaps to those within the social service profession as a whole. Rothman has also indicated, following on a number of research studies into the role of social service professionals, that 'among social work professionals, community organisers and group workers are more likely to support activist political strategies than their colleagues in casework'.[4] To the extent that community workers identify a dissonance between their values, objectives and strategies and those of their social work colleagues, they will be reluctant to make use of opportunities provided for staff development. This reluctance may derive from the apprehension that experiences such as supervision will be used to exact conformity with the department's goals and values.

The basis of the supervisor's authority
The perception of many community workers that events like supervision sessions and team meetings will be used to exact conformity with the goals and norms of the department influences and is influenced by, the community worker's view of the nature of the authority and power of those who are responsible for the management and supervision of workers. We shall explore this by using French and Raven's categories of bases of power.[5]
    They include:

coercive power (based on a capacity to withhold rewards and hand down punishments);
reward power (the provision of different kinds of rewards);
expert power (power based on knowledge and expertise);
legitimate power (that derived from legal, administrative or moral norms);
referent power (power based on personal identification with the leaders).

We believe that many community workers perceive their supervisor's authority (the supervisor is usually the Area Officer) to come largely from his higher rank in the bureaucracy (legitimate power) and partly from his power to support or refuse requests for finance for community groups (reward power).

In this kind of situation, supervisors will be seen to have both the institutional authority and the veto over financial requests that are often necessary and useful in securing compliance with the goals and norms of an agency. More significantly, many workers deny or do not acknowledge the expert and referent power of their supervisors, most of whom will be experienced in some area of casework rather than community work.

The community worker's sources of authority
The phrase 'sources of authority' is used in much the same way that it was developed by Martin Rein.[6] We use the phrase to refer to those sources from which the community worker derives authority and legitimisation for his work and activities; that is, his sanction to operate.

Rein has suggested four sources of authority for the planner, and we shall use these to indicate those of the community worker.

They are:

expertise;
bureaucratic position;
consumer preferences;
professional values.

We shall add one more source to this list:

from statute.

The authority to work of community workers in social services departments derives, whether they like it or not, from holding a position in the local authority bureaucracy, accountable to a political and administrative hierarchy. But many community workers also see themselves as accountable to the group with whom they work so that their strongest drives are to derive and assert authority as consumer advocates – as servants of community groups. We perceive this tension between *reality* (bureaucratic position) and *aspiration* (consumer advocate) as a real problem for community workers employed in social service departments.

Few workers appear to see their legitimisation deriving from one of the other three sources that are independent of the bureaucratic and advocacy positions. Community workers do not have any statutory responsibilities to their clients; we have no sense that many workers perceive themselves as subscribing to, let alone being influenced by, *professional values and goals*; and we have found that many community workers are at pains to deny that they have any claim to *expertise* from which they might derive their authority.

It may be the case that only those community workers who see their authority coming either from their expertise or bureaucratic position or from a balance of the various sources of authority will be sufficiently motivated to make use of agency-based opportunities for professional development.

The community worker's role orientation
Three basic role orientations are identifiable amongst professional workers, including those in the social services. These are:

professional orientation, where the worker is mostly influenced by the values and standards, and knowledge and methods sanctioned by a relevant professional body;
bureaucratic orientation, where the worker is influenced mostly by the policies and norms of his employing agency;
client orientation, where the worker is influenced mostly by the needs of those with whom he works.

We suggest it is a characteristic of most community workers to be firmly client-oriented, whereas various studies have shown that social workers have a high bureaucratic role orientation.[7] If community workers are aware of differences between their own and their colleagues' orientations, this may strengthen their apprehension that supervision and collegiate meetings are implicit devices for reorienting the role of the community worker towards the bureaucracy and the social work profession.

There seem to be at least two reasons why the client orientation of community workers may work against department attempts at quality control and improvement. First, community workers themselves may feel morally or politically compromised in taking up skill development opportunities from within the department. Second, their motivation to do so may be impaired; that is, recognition of the potential value of experiences like supervision may depend on community workers having a stronger orientation to their department and to a professional body.

In the remainder of the chapter we shall explore how the use by community workers of specific opportunities to develop standards of practice are affected by some of the relationships between community workers and their colleagues outlined above.

SUPERVISION

Community workers normally meet with their Area Officers in weekly or fortnightly supervision sessions – though many will not describe the sessions as supervision.[8] These meetings are perhaps the only regular occasions at which the community workers say what it is they are doing and with whom. Thus great importance should be attached to these meetings. However, most community workers attempt to treat these meetings merely as opportunities to exchange information. It is our suggestion that community workers see their weekly meetings as bounded by notions of *control* and *contamination*.

Control
Community workers are often preoccupied with their relationship to their hierarchy, and many perceive their supervision as a means of control over their activities.

   In the situation we have described the purpose of supervision ceases to be seen as that of service improvement and skill development; for many workers it rather takes on the purpose of socialising the community workers to the traditions, *mores*, values and goals of the social services, possibly with the implicit objective of weaning the worker away from his affiliation to the community workers' group and from his identification with neighbourhood groups. It may also be perceived as a way of controlling community work activities that may be politically embarrassing to the department or local authority.

Contamination
One of the major problems for anyone who has a boundary office is that of contamination. Community workers often do and say things that suggest they believe that:

they must not allow their service to the community become contaminated by their membership of, and relationships within, their departments. Thus there often seems to be a fear that they, as community workers, might become 'part of the bureaucracy';
they must not divulge information about the community to the department or area groups unless it be innocuous or harmless, in which case it does not matter.

   The concern of community workers to avoid contaminating or being contaminated by their overlapping engagement with agency and client systems may be viewed as their struggle to maintain their integrity in a situation of conflicting loyalties and commitments. This integrity is maintained by a number of devices. Some community workers, for instance, create a mystique about what it is they do. For whatever reasons, seniors or supervisors are kept at a safe distance. This is tied very much into keeping the secrets of one part of their universe (e.g. the clients) from another (e.g. their department).

Community workers will often point out, and in some cases with justification, that the skills and capacities of the Area Officer are not relevant or useful to a community worker's operations. Of course, if a community worker accepted that the Area Officer was capable and useful then it would become progressively less easy to withhold information and problems from him, and thus progressively less easy to manage the tensions of a boundary office.

The development of service competency is also hindered by the fact that community workers will often deny that they themselves are skilled workers. Emphasis is placed on 'feeling and doing' as opposed to 'thinking and knowing' and clearly such an attitude militates against successful influence by the department of *what* it is the community worker is seeking to achieve, and *how* these aims are to be achieved, and more importantly *why*.

INFORMAL DISCUSSION

Community workers may discuss their work with their community work colleagues, their social work colleagues, their managers and 'outsiders'.

Apart from those who have been caseworkers in their career, community workers tend to feel isolated in their work, and often claim that their social work colleagues do not understand what community work is about. Thus at the area level there is little talk about the job with social work colleagues. These colleagues are often seen to have a different perspective and perception of their clients. Whereas community workers see themselves as helping people to organise more effectively and develop their talents and potentials, caseworkers, it is said, see their clients in terms of problems to be defined and tackled. Outside of formal one-to-one meetings, it is not uncommon for there to be little day-to-day contact between the community worker and the Area Officer or seniors of the area group. Certainly they are not used as social workers use their team leaders, and senior managers are described as being part of the bureaucracy which is often perceived as causing the problems in the community in the first place.

IN-SERVICE COURSES AND TRAINING

Courses run by the training officers of the department to which the community worker is attached may also be seen, within the framework of control, as attempts at influence and contamination. However, very few agency-backed in-service courses seem to take place for community workers.

Where courses are run by colleges or other outside bodies a community worker will be exposed to values and *mores* which may or may not correspond to those of his department. Many community workers, however, often feel freer to talk about their work and expose themselves to new ideas outside the context of their day-to-day work.

It is important to note that for many community workers with whom we have spoken the in-service training opportunities they had taken up were, on the whole, taken up in the interests of the neighbourhood (for instance, attendance at courses to obtain knowledge about specific areas of concern to local residents, e.g. planning law and welfare rights courses). Attendance at such courses was seen as a way of transmitting relevant knowledge to community groups. The impression often given is that attendance had been discussed with the groups themselves.

USE OF CONSULTANTS

The use of outside consultants by community workers will usually depend on the availability of funds and the contacts community workers have with colleges, polytechnics, and the like. Not all authorities provide money for consultancy and, even when they do, there is often a reluctance on the part of community workers to make use of it. Those community workers who have been on courses and established contacts (usually the younger community workers) will seek consultancy, which may well provide the questioning of their work which does not take place in their department or area group. The chapter by Catherine Briscóe examines the role and function of the community work consultant.

DISCUSSION OPPORTUNITIES OUTSIDE THE AGENCY

One of the consequences of the disdain with which many community workers regard agency-based opportunities for professional self-development is that they turn to outside discussion opportunities.

Community workers often meet on their own in community workers' groups. These meetings seem to be taken up by discussion of organisational problems, particularly the individual and collective relationship of the workers to their department. The function of a community workers' group is seen more as a solidarity group – to give a sense of belonging – than a skill development or job evaluation group. This is further explored in the chapter by Peter Baldock.

Discussion with outsiders can range from wives to priests to members of community groups. Of course, workers will talk about their jobs to people they meet in social settings and the extent of such discussions is difficult to assess and perhaps not useful to know. However, discussion with community groups is important in that many community workers see this group as the only group with whom they would discuss their work problems and with whom all issues relating to them should be discussed.

However, such an approach is likely to lead the community worker even deeper into 'feeling and doing' as opposed to 'thinking and knowing' and may be detrimental to relationships with the agency and to his own competence.

CONCLUSION

A worker can learn by experience, or through working with others, or through reading on his subject. However, through experience we tend to remember unusual things and then proceed to generalise from them. It is only by an ordering of our experiences that we – community workers included – can learn from them. At present such systematic questioning does not appear to come from either the department or its community workers.

When we look at ways in which the social services department can improve service competence and develop skills, we find that the influence that it can bring to bear on its community workers is certainly limited, although of course this depends in part on the role readiness of its workers. On the whole, many community workers, by choosing with whom they should discuss the why, what and how of their work, are not exposed to any systematic influence which can monitor, assess and guide their activities.

REFERENCES

1 D. Katz and R. C. Kahn, *The Social Psychology of Organisations* (Wiley & Sons, New York, 1966), pp. 178–80.
2 For a further discussion on the differences in goals, knowledge base and strategies between community workers and those who work with individuals, families and small groups, see James K. Whittaker, *Social Treatment: An Approach to Interpersonal Helping* (Aldine Publishing Co., 1974), ch. 3.
3 The quality and techniques of role readiness are described by D. Katz and R. C. Kahn, op. cit., ch. 7. Role readiness refers to a person's anticipation of the role expectations held of him by others with whom he interacts in an organisation.
4 Jack Rothman, *Planning and Organising for Social Change* (Columbia University Press, 1974), p. 98.
5 J. R. P. French and B. Raven, 'The Bases of Social Power', in D. Cartwright and A. Zander (eds), *Group Dynamics*, 3rd edn (London Tavistock, 1968).
6 M. Rein, 'The Search for Legitimacy', *Journal of the American Institute of Planners* (July 1969).
7 See, for references, Rothman, op. cit., pp. 83–8.
8 An account of community work supervision is provided in the paper by Patrick Harris.

Chapter 2

STAFF SUPERVISION IN COMMUNITY WORK

Patrick Harris

Community work encompasses a diversity of attitudes and values. But, despite differences in philosophy and method, community workers generally see themselves as agents of social change, and they are suspicious of those in organisations, like supervisors, who seem to represent the status quo and to provide a mechanism of control over fieldworkers. Organisations employ staff to promote their aims and objectives, and they build into their administrative structures systems of accountability and control by which fieldworkers can be held responsible to decision makers. The fact that most supervisors are agency managers gives supervisory practice its administrative aspect.

Training opportunities for prospective community workers are limited and it is not essential to have a qualification to gain employment in this field. The lack of a common training experience shields workers from processes of professional socialisation inherent in the learning situation. The professional ambiance which might knit together a team of community workers with different experiences and outlooks is absent. Because of this the educational aspect of supervisory practice has a great importance. Not only will the supervisor want to increase the skills and knowledge of practitioners, but he will seek, in discussion and consultation, to encourage a common approach by the team of community workers.

Community workers often find themselves working in situations that are stressful, and they will need support that helps them understand and tolerate this stress and anxiety. Workers will also want to share problems and worries with someone who understands, yet who is sufficiently detached to comment and advise with objectivity. This is the supportive role of the community work supervisor.

Although it is useful to break down supervisory practice into three separate elements – administrative, educational and supportive – in practice they are interlocked. A fieldworker's report can be a part of a system of accountability; in its preparation the supervisor may encourage the worker to take cognisance of the value systems of those who will receive the report, which is educational; and the report may be used by a supervisor to help a fieldworker to see how his work has progressed, which is supportive. These three elements of supervisory practice are now separately considered, but the interrelatedness of the elements should be remembered.

ADMINISTRATION

Within the organisation the supervisor will have a whole or shared responsibility for the development of effective community work practice. He will contribute to the definition of aims and objectives and help evolve the necessary resources for the structure and provision of a community work service.

A supervisor is likely to be in a position to help order the community work priorities of the agency. Various factors from the practical to political will help determine priorities. A knowledge of the values of those able to influence the policy-making process, the ability to assess the relative importance of formal and informal relationships among those involved in decision making and the nature and availability of resources are among the factors a supervisor will need to consider if he is to be influential. Census data and other social indicators may also highlight areas for potential community work involvement.

If a supervisor is to maximise his effectiveness in influencing priority setting in his organisation, he needs to develop a breadth of vision and have the necessary information to operate in what are often dynamic situations. He must also have some means to structure thought and action. A supervisor should seek to develop a theoretical framework in order to link and relate activities at different operational levels. Without theoretical guidelines, a supervisor may merely react to situations rather than planning work for specific purposes.

The supervisor has a responsibility to try to create an understanding and supportive climate in which the fieldworkers can carry out their work. Whenever possible those in positions of power and influence should be made fully aware of the implications of the community work approach to be adopted. They need to be aware, for instance, that if fieldworkers assist the development of groups in the community, a group may become critical of policies of the employing organisation or be hostile to bodies whose co-operation is essential to other areas of the organisation's work. As a channel of communication the supervisor can influence those who make decisions by increasing their knowledge of community work and related matters. The use of reports and the selective involvement of influential persons are among the methods which can be used to increase knowledge. The supervisor will attempt to develop a common language and common perception of the organisation's community work task between those who exercise a management function and those in the field. The supervisor has an important role to play as a link between different organisational levels.

The failure to ensure a realistic allocation of resources to back up community workers can affect the relationship between supervisor and fieldworkers. In order to be effective, fieldworkers need relevant and adequate resources to do their job. Assistance with typing and duplicating or help with the hire of a film or a hall are the kind of servicing a community group may require. The supervisor's ability to spot under-used resources and a wider and different usage of existing provision can provide the fieldworker with the necessary flexibility and confidence to cope with changing and unpredictable situations. A resource library covering current legislation, case studies, the writings of community workers and relevant journals can be very useful. Ideally, his knowledge of the availability of resources should also help the supervisor to determine the community work priorities of the organisation.

Retaining the trust and co-operation of senior staff and fieldworkers requires a delicate and sensitive touch. A loss of support from those at the top or bottom of the hierarchy can have widespread repercussions on the provision of a community work service. Policy and decision makers can curtail or hinder the activities of community workers. Those in the field can withhold information or use a deteriorating relationship with a supervisor to act outside the constraints accepted at the time of appointment. Policy makers, senior staff and the fieldworkers will each have different expectations of the supervisor. The ability to operate effectively at the different organisational levels is an essential aspect of supervisory practice. An openness in dealings with others, a deliberate effort to help others gain an understanding of the purposes and intentions of the supervisor's tasks, and a knowledge of the values and attitudes of those to be influenced are some of the factors which can enable a supervisor to walk this administrative tightrope.

EDUCATION

The provision of an effective community work service is related to the level of skills and abilities of the fieldwork staff. The supervisor's aim is to maintain and raise the level of community work practice.

Actual experiences of fieldworkers provide the best starting place for learning and the pegs on which theory, related issues and other facts can be hung. Opportunities for discussion of practical situations will arise in formal supervisory sessions, but formal supervision, because it clearly delineates the teacher–learner roles, often inhibits community workers.

Whether a session is formal or informal, the supervisor needs background information about the fieldworker he supervises. Knowledge of the worker's background and previous experience can enable a better judgement to be made about his needs. A supervisor also seeks to understand the personal ideology or philosophy which motivates those who work with community groups. A full understanding of the community work task is necessary if the advice given is to be helpful and relevant. There is need for flexibility in the teaching role. Responding to the needs of fieldworkers may mean that the learning situation is only partially structured. Where developments are outside the experience of the supervisor and community worker, there should be a willingness to seek the help of other persons with relevant knowledge and experience.

There are two aspects of the educational component of the supervisory task – self-development and the learning of the skills and knowledge that are relevant to a fieldworker's current commitments. Both occur within the development of a theoretical framework around which supervisor and worker can organise thought and action. Such a framework can provide guidelines for action at a locality level; be the basis of co-ordinated and cohesive action between different levels of community work activity; and set out aims and objectives that can be used to monitor progress and evaluate outcomes. Without a means to structure thought and action, the service provided by the agency may lack direction and purpose. It should be remembered, however, that theory helps in understanding problems, but is not itself a source of solutions.

Self-Development

Our attitudes and responses to others are rooted in our life experience. Personal characteristics and mannerisms can directly affect a worker's attempt to establish *rapport* and a relationship with people in a community. A worker's personal preference may dictate the nature of his involvement with a group. Supervisory practice is thus concerned to explore with a fieldworker the appropriateness of his responses and actions in certain situations. In discussion a worker can be encouraged to probe his perception of 'reality' and to see whether it gives rise to actions that are an impediment to the task in which he is currently engaged. Vickers[1] has termed the perceived 'reality' of an individual, plus his values, as his 'appreciative system'. In supervision, the aim is to help a fieldworker to gain a greater awareness of his appreciative system and provide the basis for change.

Inexperienced workers may find it easier to participate in this kind of self-exploration than those with more experience. The former may appreciate that their actions may be foreign to, or offend, the cultural expectations of those in the community. An experienced worker may feel inadequate and become defensive if he is shown that many of his judgements are based on an 'appreciative system' that has shortcomings.

Skills and Knowledge

A fieldworker's active involvement in an exploration of his work is an effective way of facilitating the learning of new skills and knowledge.

Principles taught at an abstract level are far more difficult to apply than principles discovered from a person's immediate experience. By participating in analysis and interpretation, the worker will be more likely to internalise the information and values which emerge from examining his activities. When ideas that emerge from a supervisory session are a worker's own, they are more likely to be translated into practice.

Brager and Specht[2] usefully distinguish between the community worker's interactional and technical tasks. In practice a worker deals with interactional and technical tasks simultaneously and they are interrelated. Interactional tasks involve communicating with and relating to others. The identification of potential members; the motivation and recruitment of individuals into a group; the development of a group identity and cohesion; the building of a coalition with other groups; the development of leadership skills; and the achievement of necessary internal changes are some of the interactional tasks in which a community worker may become engaged.

The supervisor will encourage the community worker to notice and adapt to phases of change in the community work process. The interaction between individuals, subgroups and subcultures is another important area of consideration. Difficulties in communication between the group and its constituency, the group and resource persons in the locality, and between the worker and local people will also provide a focus for discussion in supervisory sessions.

It is important that the fieldworker keeps a written record of his work in order to provide a picture of the current situation and an insight into the thinking behind the worker's actions. By recording developments at the various stages of the community work process it is possible to review and assess the appropriateness of past actions.

It should be stressed that the participation of a community worker in a joint exploration of the work in which he is engaged is not intended to erode the concept of worker responsibility. Through the worker's involvement in the interpretation and analysis of his work he can develop increased sensitivity, a greater breadth of vision, insight, and the ability to be more flexible and responsive. At all times the supervisor is concerned to maximise the degree of discretion exercised by the fieldworker.

The technical tasks of the community worker include problem assessment, knowledge of the administrative procedures of target institutions, the ability to advise groups on planning and budgeting a project, the assessment of the resource requirements of a proposed programme and an evaluation of the undertaking. Effective community work requires fieldworkers to have substantive knowledge of particular problem areas which are the focus of community effort. Without some specialist knowledge community workers may not be able to point out the full implications of the situation affecting the community. Whether a group wants to adopt charitable status, to take action under public health legislation, participate in planning or set up a tenants' co-operative, the advice needed is of a specialist nature. Even if a resource person with the required knowledge is available on a consultative basis, the worker may still have the task of helping the community group go through each step to attain its objectives. Unless he is able to draw on very wide experience, it is not likely that a supervisor will have the range of specialist knowledge to advise and support fieldwork staff. A supervisor may tackle this in a number of different ways. Organisations have been formed as a resource to individuals and community groups. These include the National Council of Civil Liberties, the Citizens' Rights Office, the Legal Action Group and the Public Health Advisory Service. Besides providing much needed help to those seeking a solution to a problem, the organisations issue reports and case studies. A supervisor, even if he is unable to assimilate all the information, should have read enough to know what kind of information is available.

Small community work agencies may not be able to provide courses or seminars on specialist subjects for fieldwork staff. Some councils of social service and colleges of further education may be willing to put on courses, if approached. Supervisors should be actively involved, as a group, in pushing for training courses and overseeing their development.

Where an agency has a number of fieldworkers, a supervisor may be able to encourage individual community workers to develop areas of specialist knowledge. Where expertise is gathered in this way, it is essential that the information is committed to paper. Seminars conducted by those with the experience and expertise in certain problem areas are a way of communicating the difficulties and possibilities of certain kinds of action to other staff members.

Information gleaned from reports and discussions with staff can be used to provide a knowledge bank about the power structure, the value systems of those with influence, and the availability of resources. It is necessary to know in detail the procedures and the mode of practice of the local council. For instance, a fieldworker should be able to advise a community group on how to put in a request for a local authority to receive a delegation, and also on how the delegation is likely to be received. In the compilation of a directory of local intelligence the supervisor has a co-ordinating and facilitating role. Where an assessment has to be made as to the tactics and strategies open to community groups, the supervisor's responsibility is to ensure that the relevant knowledge and information about the local situation is available.

SUPPORTIVE ROLE

Long, demanding hours, the need to work in an unstructured situation, the tensions inherent in conflict strategies, and feelings of despondency because there appears to be no observable progress are some of the sources of pressure experienced by the community worker. If an individual is subject to constant psychological stress, his effectiveness as a worker will be lessened. The supportive element of supervisory practice is thus concerned with helping practitioners to cope with or reduce pressures.

A supervisory session can act as a safety valve, providing an opportunity for feelings of frustration and anger to be vented. A fieldworker may find himself having to offer words of encouragement to community groups when things go wrong and to hide his own disappointment. When this happens, a supervisor may have to be a good listener, helping the worker to interpret his experience in a positive way.

Long, unsocial hours can make neighbourhood workers feel jaded and worn out. The use and allocation of time should therefore be subject to periodic review at supervision sessions. When a community's activities have developed a recognisable pattern, it is relatively easy for community workers to develop a habitual response. A supervisor can encourage a fieldworker to consider whether his involvement is really necessary and to question whether the most effective use is being made of his skill and energies.

Those involved on a day-to-day basis in a locality are sometimes too close to the action to notice gradual change over a period of time. In such circumstances, a fieldworker may have doubts about the value of his work and his own abilities. Written records can be used to chart developments both within a group and in its external relations. Knowledge of achievements arising from community work practice may not only serve to dispel feelings of despondence but may also encourage a worker to raise his sights when confronted with the outcome of his efforts.

When a mistake is made, it is necessary to find out why it occurred. If the fieldworker happens to be the wrong man for the job, then efforts should be made to determine his strengths and to involve him in work to which they are relevant. If the mistake is due to inexperience or a poor analysis of the situation, steps have to be taken to reduce the possibility of a recurrence. At the same time, the supervisor needs to make it clear that the worker still has his confidence. An error of judgement can set the community work process back and the worker's belief in himself may be shaken. It is important that the community worker is given every opportunity to find a solution in a manner which restores the worker's sense of purpose and removes feelings of self-doubt.

SOME PROBLEMS IN SUPERVISION

The elements of supervisory practice have been set out above. The principles of community work supervision have not been related to the actual situations and difficulties faced by supervisors in their work. Problems peculiar to the employing organisation, the lack of relevant experience of the supervisor, or conflict of views and ideas with fieldwork staff may be a source of difficulties for the supervisor.

The employing agency

In large organisations the role of community workers may be perceived differently by persons at various levels of the hierarchy. Terms of reference are often phrased in such general terms that they are open to a range of interpretations. A community work supervisor is the guardian of the practitioner's definition of the terms of reference and he has an educative role in relation to those who exercise influence and power. Where the practitioner's definition is not fully accepted, the supervisor and community workers will have to frame reports and requests for resources in a manner acceptable to those who make the decisions. In a social services department, for example, it is necessary to relate community work activities to social work aims and objectives. If community work is seen to be peripheral to the main purposes of the organisation, there is likely to be a lack of support and a reluctance to commit resources to it. A supervisor will seek to maximise the community work influence on the policy-making processes, but at the same time to maintain the integrity of community work practice.

Problems of differing expectations of community work are found also in non-hierarchical organisations. Individual groups in a consortium, such as a federation of tenants' associations, may perceive the community worker's role differently. Members or member groups need to be encouraged to discuss community work and develop a common perception of community work objectives and methods.

The recognition of organisational constraints does not debar a supervisor (or fieldworkers) from seeking to change the nature of these constraints. Legitimate channels exist through which organisational change can be sought, though some, such as trade unions and professional organisations, are sometimes overlooked. The rules, procedures and methods of organisations are instruments to achieve certain purposes. They are not sacrosanct and a supervisor should seek to instigate and participate in organisational change in order to protect and promote community work interests.

The lack of relevant experience of those with a supervisory role

A problem which is found far too frequently in social work agencies is the delegation of supervisory responsibility for community workers to persons without any previous practical experience in community work. This is most frequently found in social service departments, in which community workers have often been attached to area offices and the supervisory role has fallen to a senior social worker or area officer. Whilst a supervisor without relevant practical experience may be able to cope with the administrative element of his role, he has not the skills or knowledge necessary to tackle the educational or supportive elements. The high turnover of community work staff in social service departments is in part a result of the inadequacy of the supervision provided.

Outside consultants or advisers can be employed to remedy the deficiencies. The problem, however, must be recognised before such appointments can be made. Supervisors may be invited to join local community workers' groups, where they exist. Special training programmes should be put on for prospective supervisors and their problems examined and discussed. The use of consultants, the involvement of supervisors in local community workers' groups, and training for supervisors can improve the situation but cannot be as effective as supervision by an experienced community worker.

Where no attempt is made to develop the necessary supervisory skills, the supervisor may lose credibility in the eyes of the fieldwork staff. If a supervisor feels threatened and forced on the defensive, he may fall back on the body of knowledge which has been the basis of earlier professional practice. Instead of giving support the supervisor can then become the source of new pressures on the fieldworker. Those concerned with training need to tackle the problem of how to increase the effectiveness of supervisors, who are failing to provide the level of supervision required. The attitudes of senior staff members assigned to carry out community work supervision are important. Do they give high priority to supervisory responsibilities? Are they prepared to develop the necessary knowledge and skills? If the right attitudes exist and the right educational input is provided in training, the standards of community work supervision can be raised.

The fieldworker

Idealism is a quality often found among community workers. It has its advantages and disadvantages. It is important that those concerned with social change have a belief in their cause. On the other hand, idealism may impede realistic analysis and thus reduce the effectiveness of the worker.

Many fieldworkers (and supervisors) will obtain sanction for their actions from philosophies and ideologies outside the employing agency. There can be conflict between the community worker's ideology and that of the organisation which employs him. The possibility of conflict can be reduced if the constraints of the organisation are spelt out to the prospective community worker at the time of the interview for the post. A condition of employment should be the willingness of a worker to operate within the constraints. Recognition and acceptance does not take away the right of the worker to seek to change the nature of the constraints.

Major difficulties occur when a community worker chooses to act outside the constraints of the organisation. The actions of one worker can impose restrictions on his colleagues. A supervisor can use coercive powers against a worker but in doing so he can lose the co-operation, information and help a fieldworker is able to provide. If the constraints and methods of an agency have been explained to a worker prior to his taking up a post, these can be the basis of his employment and he can be prevailed upon to act within them.

Disagreement between the community worker and his supervisor about the worker's values and activities often highlights the role of the supervisor as an agent of social and organisational control. Indeed, many supervisors feel they have a responsibility to help community workers to develop principles and standards of practice that are within the norms and goals of their agency and profession. They may disagree with a particular strategy, like a rent strike, or with the involvement of local people in alternative institutions and fringe political parties. They may disagree with the political views of the community worker, or with his life and work styles, and suspect that he is using the local community as a test-bed for his own social and political beliefs.

The primary loyalty of many community workers is to those in the community with whom they work. A supervisor has to understand this loyalty, but not necessarily to share it. A community worker's commitment is often to a particular group or neighbourhood, but that of a supervisor is to a more effective agency service, including more effective community work. In the final analysis, however, a supervisor should strive to help his community workers become more independent, self-critical and self-directing.

REFERENCES

1 Sir Geoffrey Vickers, *Value Systems and Social Process* (Tavistock Publications, 1968).
2 George Brager and Harry Specht, *Community Organizing* (Columbia University Press, 1973).

FURTHER READING

Dorothy E. Pettes, *Supervision in Social Work* (George Allen & Unwin, 1967).

Chapter 3

THE CONSULTANT IN COMMUNITY WORK

Catherine Briscoe

With the upsurge of interest in community work in Britain in the late 1960s and early 1970s, numbers of community work positions have been created in organisations where supervisory and managerial staff have little knowledge of the practice or problems of this field. In consequence experienced community workers from other fields and community work teachers are increasingly being asked for help and advice as consultants both for the community worker and for his agency.

Four different patterns of such consultancy seem to be emerging.

The earliest form developed in the 1960s with the growth of experimental community work projects founded by trusts and with advisory and/or executive committees, composed of representatives from a variety of voluntary and statutory organisations. Consultants in these projects were an integral part of the structure and usually were present at advisory or executive committee meetings. They gave help both to the workers in the project and to the committee in planning and developing its work. George Goetschius has described his role as a consultant to one such project.[1]

Community workers are also employed in a variety of settings which, unlike the experimental projects, are not primarily focused on community work. Social service departments, planning departments, voluntary agencies and other organisations have employed community workers often as the only worker within that organisation performing the particular functions of community work. These workers and their employing agencies have developed the three other patterns of consultancy to provide support in the performance of community work tasks.

The second form has arisen where community workers from a variety of settings have taken the initiative, come together as a group and invited consultants to be present at the meetings of the group and to work with them on a variety of subjects.

Third, community workers within one agency have also invited consultants to meet with them to discuss the particular work in which they are involved. Such an invitation may be given by the community worker(s) direct to the consultant, by the agency at the worker's request, or by the agency as a provision offered to the community worker prior to his employment. Such consultancy may be offered to each community worker individually or to a group of workers employed in the same agency.

The fourth form of consultancy is the most recent and appears to be developing as agencies become more aware of the needs of their staff for help. This is the employing of consultants as members of staff of an organisation, a department, or of a local authority. Community work consultants or advisers in social service departments, for instance, are responsible both for offering support and help to community workers and for promoting and developing community work activities within the department.

In each of these forms of consultancy, the consultant is invited to offer his help either to a group, an individual or an agency as a whole around the community work aspects of its service. For the consultant there are, however, basic dilemmas in defining what is expected of him in the consultant role.

First, the consultant may be called in to supplement agency provisions for community workers in supervision, training, management and/or peer group support. As described later he may be asked to help in a considerable variety of ways. Second, consultants are chosen for their experience and knowledge of community work and are requested to put these at the service of their consultees. They rarely have training in consultancy, and, while there is literature on consultancy in fields such as mental health and education which can be helpful, there is little to give guidance on the objectives or the process of consultancy specific to community work. Third, agencies that have found difficulty in defining the task of the community worker (cf. the chapter by Thomas and Warburton) are even less able to define how the community work consultant should be used. The community worker may be aware of needing help, but can rarely be explicit about the kind of help he needs. Thus the consultant has the task of defining for himself the objectives and the particular tasks of his role in whatever consultancy situation he finds himself. This definition can only be based on his understanding of:

what he himself has to offer;
what kind of help is being requested in the consultancy into which he is being invited.

THE INVESTMENT OF THE CONSULTANT

The consultant has expectations concerning what he will put into consultation and what he himself will gain from it.[2] He usually has had experience in the field, may or may not have had training in community work, and may or may not have been in a position to study, conceptualise, teach or write about community work. He will bring to consultancy knowledge and skills developed from experience and/or training and study, his own ideas as to what constitutes good community work practice, and an interest in the promotion of community work activities.

In addition, the consultant brings a detachment from the day-to-day problems of both the agency and the community work activity which enables him to look at alternatives without being under pressure to make instant decisions. He also brings a certain amount of time and energy, though at the moment these are limited, at least for external consultants, since few community work consultants are in a position to make consultancy a recognised part of their job description and allocate to it any substantial amount of their working time.

Given the limitations on time and energy of the consultant, consultation must hold certain attractions, apart from purely financial ones. These include:

1 a wish on the part of community work teachers to keep in touch with the field;
2 an interest in trying out ideas and concepts developed through study;
3 an investment in developing the field and helping practitioners improve their knowledge and skills;
4 a personal investment in the promotion of community work;
5 an interest in helping others avoid mistakes one may have made oneself, or seen others make.

Whatever the consultant's interest in the particular situation he is always conscious of being there by invitation only, even as an internal consultant. Consultees will use his advice and help at their own volition as he normally has little power to enforce his suggestions.

TYPES OF HELP REQUESTED

Practitioners and/or their agencies ask for help around a considerable diversity of subjects including planning, training, problem clarification, conflict mediation and confirming values and goals.[3]

1 *Planning*

Initial planning. In experimental projects the consultant was usually involved in planning for the project as a whole, as he was likely to be one of the few people available to the advisory/executive committee, and to the worker, who had any knowledge of what might be appropriate goals and structures for community work activities. As the internal or external consultant to workers from one agency, the consultant may be invited to participate in the initial design of community work within an agency.

This happens where the agency and/or the community worker recognise the need for such clarification to take place, and undertake to plan for the development of community work activities. Consultants are requested to help the agency and the worker choose and define possible objectives in the light of:

a the goals of the agency and the services it offers which will determine in part the type of relationship it requires with the community;[4, 5]
b the situation of and the needs felt by people in the particular 'community', be it a given locality or a specified population group.

Such a determination of priorities gives both the agency and the new worker a clearer idea of his initial focus and of the issues within the community which he will emphasise in his own initial assessment and study. It clarifies the kinds of support and resources the worker will need from the agency to develop his activities according to the plan. It also helps to clarify both for the worker and for his agency what kind of information the agency requires from the worker in order to provide him with backing. The consultant involved in planning goals and priorities can, ideally, help both agency and worker understand the implications and mutual demands of the contract they establish.

Ongoing planning. Planning where community workers are already involved in various activities is also a focus of consultation discussions. Even experienced community workers can find consultancy helpful in considering alternatives of action at different stages of their work and in looking at the potential contribution of such action to the long- and short-term goals of the worker, the action system and the employing agency.

2 Training
In most agencies there is some provision for in-service training or other professional development for staff. As described by Thomas and Warburton Chapter 1, community workers often have problems in taking up the opportunities provided by their agencies. Both agencies and community workers look to consultants as trainers, and expect help in the improvement of practice and the development of ongoing work. The task of the consultant in training is to identify the particular areas of difficulty which interfere with the consultee's ability to perform. Lack of knowledge and understanding, lack of skill, lack of objectivity and lack of confidence and self-esteem are areas identified by Caplan[6] as blockages for those working in the mental health field. Community workers often seem to face similar blockages though the context is different and the range of factors to be taken into account in community work are normally more diverse.

Lack of knowledge and understanding is most acute among untrained community workers but it is felt by all practitioners faced with a job which is invariably complex and demanding. Consultees may be unaware of a whole range of factors which affect their tasks, such as the processes of group life, techniques of doing surveys, sources of information for community assessments, and many others. Consultation on an individual basis is an uneconomic way of teaching basic information and consultants are often alert to the possibility of short courses or seminars in which consultees can participate to acquire such training more intensively. With groups of consultees from the same agency, or from a variety of settings, it is possible to identify the most important gaps in group members' knowledge, and to work out a group agenda for discussion. The consultant often needs to bring in other resources for seminars of this nature, such as lawyers, planners and other specialists.

Lack of skill affects the ability of the worker to use himself and to make choices in any situation. For instance, he may have difficulty in seeing how to behave with members of his action system or with colleagues and seniors. A common question from consultees is: 'Should I take the initiative in suggesting action or should I wait for members of the action system to bring out their own ideas?'

The consultant helps the consultee consider the given situation and recognise the factors involved and their relative importance. In the above example these might include the stage of development of the action system, the experience of the various members in working on the issue concerned and the information on this issue available to the worker. As the consultee gains experience in considering choices his own skill in making them develops.

Lack of objectivity is a difficulty for community workers, since they must work with a variety of people, differing in personal characteristics and points of view. Dislike of, disagreement with, or ideological bias against key figures in action and target systems, or in the consultee's own agency, can block the ability to understand their motivations and resistance to change. The consultee, even if he has knowledge and skill, may be unable to use these if he cannot get past his personal reactions. For instance, a community worker who works with an elderly, domineering chairman of a community group may find himself devoting his energy to a palace revolution within the group, and unable to help the group as a whole to work towards its defined goal, whatever that may be. If the consultee feels the consultant to be sympathetic to his own feelings the consultant can help the consultee look at why his own reactions to the chairman are so strong and if those reactions are shared by other members of the group or of the community they represent. Together they can look at the contributions of the chairman, the other group members and the consultee to the overall goals of the group and choose a plan of action related to the achievement of those goals.

Lack of confidence and self-esteem can arise from such factors as fatigue, frustration, opposition, or just from inexperience on the part of the worker. It can interfere with his job performance, making him hesitant in presenting himself and his ideas to the variety of people with whom he works. The consultant can help with encouragement and acceptance of the consultee, but must do this tactfully or the consultee may feel patronised and even less confident.

In the training aspects of his task, the consultant may encounter particular problems. Community workers hold conflicting views about training, its value and its desirability. Some members of a group, or even individual consultees whose agencies have directed them towards the consultant for training, may feel that the identification of knowledge and skills needed for the performance of community work is immoral and places the practitioner at too great a remove from the community. Where the consultant encounters this belief in individual consultees he is blocked in offering training. Where some members of a group hold such views it is difficult to continue discussion with the other members and perhaps the consultancy pattern must be altered.

As well as those conflicts around training which are peculiar to community work the consultant will also meet the individual responses of consultees as adult learners to the process of changing behaviour and developing new attitudes through new learning. If the consultant is involved in helping the consultee acquire knowledge and skill to improve his job performance, he will also be involved in helping the consultee cope with his own ambivalence about acknowledging the need for change and actually utilising what he learns.

Where the consultant is part of the management of the agency, this particular difficulty may be compounded by the consultee's feelings about authority and by the consultant's sense of responsibility towards the agency and its clientele. Community workers tend to be suspicious of 'contamination' (cf. Thomas and Warburton, Chapter 1) and of control by their agency, and may suspect that the consultant has been co-opted into the agency establishment. This will increase resistance to integrating learning gained through consultancy. The consultant in his concern for the agency's programme, and with the need to win greater acceptance and more resources for community work within the agency, may himself find difficulties in allowing a community worker to use learning and develop work in his own way, which may be dissimilar to that of the consultant.

3 Problem Clarification
The consultant is often invited to help with a specific problem which

consultees are experiencing in their work. Such problems may, for example, be related to the complexity of a particular issue which has arisen in a community, such as a redevelopment plan where the consultee and/or his agency are uncertain as to what steps to take; they may be related to conflicts between differing groups in the community; or they may arise out of determined efforts by target systems to stop or control the activity of community groups or workers. The consultant is asked to focus on the specific problem, to discover what is involved and to help consultees to remove, get around, or solve the problem. In this form of help, the consultant must look outside the consultee and his agency at the action systems and target systems with which the consultee is involved. Concentrated time and effort is required over a short period of time.

The status and experience of the consultant can be of importance in this type of consultancy in gaining access to key figures in local government or in opposing groups. It is also easier for an external consultant to approach key figures involved in the problem where the conflict is between them and the consultee and/or consultee agency. Problems the consultant is likely to find in giving this kind of help include possible resistance on the part of the consultee and/or his agency to findings which show a need for change on their part[7] and the handling of information shared with him confidentially in the course of his investigation which seems important to communicate to consultees in justifying the proposals for change.

4 *Conflict mediation*
This form of consultancy resembles problem clarification closely both in process and in the sort of difficulties the consultant is likely to encounter in carrying it out. The separate term is used to denote situations where help is requested in conflicts between community workers and their employers. Examples of such conflicts might be where a new senior staff member has been appointed who has different priorities for community work activities from those of the community worker who worked in agreement with his predecessor, or where groups with which the worker is involved have become actively critical of the employing or funding agency, or of other departments within a local authority.

In such situations the worker may be looking for support and help in changing the attitudes of his agency while the agency may be looking to the consultant to 'tame' the community worker and teach him better practice.

The task of the consultant as in problem clarification is to attempt to gain information as to the sources of the conflict and then to negotiate proposals with each party for its solution. Here the internal consultant who has a recognised role towards the advisory/executive committee or management group and who is regarded as being a consultant to both parties is often in a better position to gather such information and to help conflicting parties to determine where the conflict lies. While each of the conflicting parties may try to co-opt him to their side, he is recognised by both the community worker and the agency to have some responsibility for ensuring the continuation of both the agency and the community work service. Perhaps the consultant may be involved in pushing agency staff and executives to take a more understanding and supportive stance towards community work. At other times, the consultant might suggest the community worker should think more of the needs of his employing agency. The consultant is involved in helping each to recognise the needs of the other and in improving communication and co-operation between the two.

The external consultant may find it more difficult to be accepted in the mediating role. Frequently, the community worker is seen as the consultee of the external consultant and the agency does not recognise any particular role for the consultant vis-a-vis its own structure and policy. Even where the consultant is asked for advice or intervention, his identification with community work may cause him to be seen by both the worker and the agency as 'on the worker's side' and not as an impartial participant.

5 Confirming Values and Goals

Community workers may often meet with lack of interest or even active opposition from other staff members. They will then tend to search for like-minded people outside the agency who will help them confirm *the legitimacy and worth of their goals and values*. Consultants from outside the agency, whether invited to consult with a group or with individual workers, are often seen as providing both confirmation of legitimacy and worth and, by virtue of their experience and position, a degree of status for community work activities. Consultants employed within the agency may offer more in this particular aspect since they are a visible sign of the agency's recognition of community work, and, by virtue of their position, offer status and a voice within management for community work priorities and goals. This is primarily an emotional response of the consultee to the presence of the consultant rather than one based on something the consultant does, and it may or may not be recognised by the consultee and consultant. It is rarely seen as a prime objective of consultancy, but as a part of the consultancy relationship. Its presence as a factor in consultancy relationships can intensify difficulties of disagreement about goals, values and action between consultant and consultee. The consultee can find himself in conflict with someone he had perceived as 'on his side'. It can be extremely difficult for consultants and consultees who place priorities on difference change objectives to work together if these differences are not clearly acknowledged and understood. Each may be working towards his own goals from the basis of different perspectives on society, and therefore be looking towards totally different tactics and strategies.[8]

The consultee may find this disagreement difficult to cope with in the light of his need for confirmation and support. The consultant may also find this conflict difficult. For example, the consultant may perceive himself as having moved, in the course of his experience in community work, from broad-sweeping goals of change in the structure of society to a more realistic and limited view of what is actually possible. If the consultee represents the kind of idealism from which the consultant has moved, the consultant may have to cope with a sense of guilt, with defensiveness at his own alteration and/or with impatience at the 'naivety' of the consultee, who has not experienced his own frustrations. The consultee may perceive the consultant as having been corrupted by age and/or status into supporting the status quo. Alternatively, the consultant may, from his experience and study, be convinced about the need for far-reaching changes in the structure of society, and may be confronted with the consultee's belief in limited goals related to service delivery or local self-help groups. The consultant in this situation may be perceived by the consultee as being too far removed from the struggles of the actual job to recognise limits and of being so intent on structural change that he ignores the immediate needs of community residents.

THE PROCESS OF CONSULTATION

The consultant who is involved in different consultations gradually begins to develop a format for himself which attempts to avoid some of the problems concerned and to take into account the still confused state of the community field work. Each person's format or checklist in starting a consultation will be ideal rather than actual. A checklist for consultancy might look something like this:

1 *Initial Exploration after the Request for Consultancy*
Time should be taken in the early stages of consultancy for discussions with all those involved in both the community work activity as a whole and in the specific request for consultancy. These discussions would include community workers, their immediate colleagues, supervisors and others in the management of the agency as appropriate and would cover:

the kind of help each thinks is necessary and the nature of the problem as each perceives it;
the goals and priorities each has established for community work; the extent to which these have been thought through, and the extent to which verbal and written agreement among all concerned has been reached on them;
the resources which are available for community work on the part of the practitioner and his employing agency, e.g. training, experience, finance, administrative and secretarial support, etc.

the resources which everyone involved (including the consultant) is willing to put into the consultancy, e.g. time, meeting space, priority of concentration, written material such as records, reports or committee minutes, finance.

During this preliminary phase, it is important to discuss the consultant's own view of community work, his investment in consultation and his resources of experience and study with all concerned so that they may judge the suitability of the consultant for their needs, just as he will be making judgements on their suitability for what he has to offer.

This preliminary exploration is vital and the consultant or the consultees may well decide to withdraw after this phase. The initial discussion of goals, priorities and help sought may offer both the worker(s) and the agency sufficient clarification for them to work together without the consultant. It may demonstrate that a different form of help is needed, such as courses on specific skills or knowledge areas. It may simply show that the ideas of community work of the worker(s), the agency and the consultant are so incompatible that they cannot work together.

If, however, some potential for continuing consultancy seems to be shown by this exploration, the next important point would be the agreement on contract.

2 Contract Establishing

The consultant should attempt to get agreement from all those involved, if possible in writing, on the following aspects:

the focus and goals of the consultancy. That is, is the purpose to plan activity? Is it to train practitioners? Etc. It may be advisable to recognise that more than one purpose may be involved and the focus should not be too limited.
the manner of the consultancy: whether it is to be individual or group sessions; whether there will be seminars, discussions from written materials etc.
those who will participate and their different roles: how will the content of the consultancy be related to others involved but not present, such as colleagues and immediate seniors?
the tasks to be undertaken by each participant, e.g. reports and records to be written, agenda preparation, meetings to be arranged;
a time-limit to be set for reporting and evaluation, so that after a specified period of time there is an opportunity to discuss progress and mutual satisfaction and to negotiate a revision of the contract if that seems appropriate.

A contract statement should be negotiated between all the parties involved in and affected by the consultancy, and should be available in written form as a point of reference.

Problems often arise in the course of consultancy between consultants, community workers and their agencies where a contract agreement has not been clearly developed. They may come from:

difference in expectations about the goals and purposes of the consultation; inadequate preliminary analysis of the causes of difficulties, which leads to the consultant and consultee working, for instance, on training questions rather than on conflict of priorities within the agency;

disagreements about control and accountability over such questions as the use of a worker's records or the access of the consultant to members of community groups;

incomplete contracts where the consultant and consultee have entered upon consultation without involving the consultee's immediate colleagues or seniors in prior discussion.

3 *The Process of Consultancy*

It is more difficult to suggest check-points for the actual consultancy process since this depends largely on the relationship established between consultant, consultee and the consultee's employing agency. However, there are some aspects of which the consultant can be aware and with which he can work:

recognising and thinking about resistance and motivations to change and attempting to work in ways which help consultees accept and integrate new learning. Literature on adult education and on supervision in social work can offer some help here;[9, 10]

if working with a group, trying to develop an open relationship with and between group members so that workers know the position and perspective of each other and of the consultant. New members coming into the group need introductions and orientation to the group from the consultant or from other members so that they are aware of the agreed contract and can participate on that basis, withdraw from the group or attempt to re-negotiate the contract.

the consultant must bear in mind the environment of the consultancy and, even if the relationship with others involved has been settled in the contract, he should check periodically on the reactions of colleagues, supervisors and others affected;

the consultant should try to help all parties keep to the terms of the contract, pointing out where deviations have occurred. Obvious blocks may arise which necessitate renegotiation, but it is all too easy to be distracted to alternative topics or to let agreements, for example on written work, lapse. The goal of the consultancy would then be defeated or at least not fully achieved. Obviously, the consultant must be meticulous in fulfilling his own obligations under the contract;

the consultant must be aware of his own biases and attempt not to force his views on consultee(s). The consultant who is committed to community work and to his own way of working may find it very difficult to help consultees make their own choices and develop their own plan of action. It may be helpful here to consider the similarities between the consultancy process and the community work process, particularly the non-directive model offered by Batten, working from where the 'client'/consultee is helping them 'decide for themselves what their needs are: what, if anything, they are willing to do to meet them; and how they can best organise, plan, and act to carry their project through'.[11]

4 Evaluation and Feedback

Reports and discussions which are developed on evaluation and feedback should allow the consultant and consultee to summarise their perceptions of the consultancy, its usefulness to them and recommendations for its continuance, termination or renegotiation. A written report can also be a useful tool to present findings on problems and possibilities identified during the course of the consultation. These findings can be shared with the employing agency and with others whom the parties to the consultancy may wish to influence. In developing such a report, and in going through the evaluation process, consultant and consultee should consider who else should be involved in the process and with whom they may wish to share their findings.

CONCLUSIONS

The role of the community work consultant, like that of the community workers, is complex and at present relatively undefined. The consultant has the task of setting his own boundaries in deciding what he is willing and able to offer in a consultancy service. Given the present state of the community work field and the needs both of agencies and practitioners for help in such a diversity of areas, it is difficult for the consultant to say that this or this is not an appropriate consultancy task but one which should be performed by a supervisor or a trainer. Such staff are not widely available for community work. However, the consultant's understanding of the shortages in the field and his interest in promoting community work may lead him to overstretch himself and/or agree to provide service where it is inappropriate. He may feel some hesitancy, if his community work attitudes of response to expressed needs inhibit him, in exploring more fully the requests made to him and in pushing for clear terms of agreement which he negotiates with consultees and consultee agencies.

However, consultancy is a way of promoting and improving community work practice. By exploring the situation of the practitioner and/or the agency prior to setting a contract, and by then establishing clear terms of reference, the consultant is already placing himself in the advocate role for community work. He is demonstrating clearly his own view of community work as an activity which requires prior thought and planning, setting of goals and priorities, and the commitment of resources. For both the agency and the workers involved the consultant is providing a model for the establishment of a programme.

He is also, where required, making sure that he can justify to his own agency or employer the expenditure of his own time and resources upon the consultancy task.

REFERENCES

1 George Goetschius, 'Role of the Consultant', in Derek Cox (ed.), *A Community Approach to Youth Work in East London* (Y.W.C.A., 1970).
2 For further discussion on this see Ronald Lippitt, 'Dimensions of the Consultant's Job', in Kramer and Specht (eds), *Readings in Community Organization Practice* (Prentice Hall, New Jersey, 1969).
3 For detailed categorisation of consultant roles see David Macarov, *'A Study of the Consultation Process'* Part III (State Communities Aid Association, New York, 1968).
4 Violet Sieder, 'The Community Organization of the Direct Service Agency', in Kramer and Specht (eds), *Readings in Community Organization Practice* (Prentice Hall, New Jersey, 1969).
5 Catherine Briscoe, 'Community Work in Social Service Departments', *Social Work Today* (15th April, 1976).
6 Gerald Caplan, *The Theory & Practice of Mental Health Consultation* (Tavistock Publications, 1970).
7 Charles T. McElvaney and Matthew B. Miles, 'Using Survey Feedback & Consultation', in Schmuck and Miles (eds), *Organization Development in Schools* (Palo Alto, California National Press, 1971).
8 George Brager and Harry Specht, *Community Organizing* (Columbia Press, New York, 1973), p. 263.
9 For example, Leland P. Bradford, 'The Teaching-Learning Transaction' in *Adult Education*, Vol. 8, No. 3, 1958 (Adult Education Association, Chicago); Jennier Rogers, *Adults Learning* (Penguin Books, 1971).
10 For example, Lola G. Selby, 'Helping Students in Field Practice Identify and Modify Blocks to Learning', in Younghusband (ed.), *Education for Social Work*, National Institute for Social Work Training Series, No. 4 (George Allen & Unwin Ltd, London, 1968).
11 Thomas R. Batten, *The Non-Directive Approach in Group & Community Work* (Oxford University Press, London, 1967), chap. 2.

FURTHER READING

Fritz Steele, *Consulting for Organizational Change* (University of Massachusetts Press, 1975).

Chapter 4

THE COMMUNITY WORKERS' GROUP AND TRAINING

Peter Baldock

One of the primary characteristics of community work at the present moment is that the worker is often subjected to a degree of isolation in the job. He has very little in the way of institutionalised professional support and is likely to have relatively little support within his own agency. 'Bureaucracy' is already a dirty word and 'professional' is becoming one in some circles. For many the attraction of community work is precisely its relative freedom from institutional entanglements which, they feel, allows a better response to the people with whom they are working. Nevertheless, the absence of professional and agency support is a source of strain as well as of freedom of action. It is for this reason that many community workers have sought support from colleagues through the vehicle of groups of community workers meeting on a regular basis. That such groups were felt to be needed is demonstrated by the fact that the setting up of one has usually followed close on the establishment of a number of community work posts in an area. Most of the big cities have had them since 1971.

Community workers' groups have been created because a need has been felt. But the exact nature of that need is still very ill-defined. It is not merely that the groups vary among themselves as to what their function should be, but that in most of the groups taken individually there is no clear conception of function. At first glance the groups may seem similar to each other. But they vary in several ways, and one of the most crucial of these is in composition.

THE COMPOSITION OF GROUPS

A few groups have restricted membership to those they consider to be community workers. This raises the spectre of professionalism but, in fact, such groups define 'community worker' in terms of work done rather than qualifications. The Community Development Information Group in Liverpool, which is such a group, included at one time a number of people barred from full membership of the Association of Community Workers on grounds of lack of qualification. Other community workers' groups have accepted members on the basis that they define themselves as community workers and this is probably true of most of the groups. Such a procedure has the apparent advantage of not being elitist. But the advantage is a dubious one. An initial decision has to be made as to who should be invited to the first meeting and this carries an implicit decision as to the type of group composition needed. The form of composition that goes farthest in avoiding elitism is that in which membership is open to anyone interested in community work (as opposed to anyone who thinks he actually does it). The Manchester group has tended to work on this basis and, besides community workers, has attracted from time to time interested social workers, clergy, community relations officers, students, Parks Department officials and others. It has, indeed, gone out of its way to include people who are not community workers when issues relating to their field are under discussion.

These different types of composition involve more than different types of people. They also effect the extent to which the group is a coherent one. Evidently, the group with the more restricted membership, provided that such a group is felt to be useful by its potential members, is more likely to have a strong group feeling and some consistency of operation. The group which defines its potential membership loosely is likely to have a large and changing one, making effective action or even discussion over a period difficult.

THE ORGANISATION OF MEETINGS

Variations in composition are matched by variations in the organisation of meetings. A monthly meeting summoned on a regular date by a secretary or convener is the most common form. Even within the framework of the monthly meeting there are variations of organisational detail with more informality in the organisation of some groups than of others. Moreover, the monthly meeting can have two quite different purposes. Members may opt for regular and comparatively frequent meetings to ensure continuity of operation and thereby make it easier for the group to undertake seriously some course of action or discussion. Alternatively, the regular monthly meeting may be selected to make it easier for people to remember when meetings are taking place and thus facilitate casual attendance at them. This may help to ensure that a larger number of people are kept in the network whose formal basis is the group.

Some groups have recognised that monthly meetings are seen in different ways by different members and have attempted to set up different forms of meeting for the purposes of organised discussion on the one hand and casual contact on the other. The Sheffield group, for example, experimented with a system under which Friday lunchtime at a particular pub was chosen as a regular weekly casual meeting point for community workers at which information could be exchanged. It was anticipated that general issues arising out of discussion at these informal pub sessions could be made the subject of organised meetings for those interested in them. This system broke down very rapidly. The weekly pub session rarely seemed sufficiently attractive for people to make a special journey from where they were working to the pub concerned. In the absence of the informal contacts supposedly provided by the pub sessions it was impossible to organise the meetings on special interests. Within six months the monthly meetings had recommenced.

THE TASKS OF COMMUNITY WORKERS' GROUPS

Variety in relation to composition and organisation is closely connected to variety in the tasks undertaken by the groups. Logically, the functions of a group should be defined first. These will suggest a number of tasks. The tasks should define the composition and organisation needed. In practice this order has been reversed. Because of the way the groups have been set up in response to an often vaguely felt need, the tasks and therefore possible functions have been selected largely on the basis of the sort of meetings that have evolved. Exchange of hard local information has been the most common task and in the more coherent groups this has led to forms of co-ordinated action. One of the interesting things about the groups in that very few of the tasks frequently undertaken relate to professional development or training.

VARIATIONS IN RELATIONSHIP WITH ACW

The three variations so far mentioned seem to me the most important, but variations in the amount of contact with the Association of Community Workers are also significant. I leave the Community and Youth Service Association to one side because it does have a branch structure of its own, though one essentially geared to the youth rather than community aspect of CYSA's concerns. ACW still lacks any branch structure and it is the presence of the local community workers' groups that has inhibited the development of such a structure, since ACW has wished to avoid appearing to make a takeover. The members of the local groups who play a most active part in them are usually ACW members and the ACW members have sometimes met in *ad hoc* local sessions, usually to prepare for the Association's AGM. The absence of a formal link between ACW and the local groups damages the work of both. The local groups really are local. Lacking any formal link with a national body they find it difficult to influence national policy even on such matters as training and conditions of employment. In fact, few of the groups appear to have considered such issues within their range. ACW, lacking any real base and too low in resources for adequate contact to be maintained with the individual members, may keep in touch with opinion among fieldworkers, but lacks the credibility and strength to pursue many matters forcefully enough to have an effect.

THE POSSIBILITY OF A TRAINING FUNCTION

I have outlined at comparative length the present nature of the local community workers' groups because I wish to bring out clearly two points that have a major bearing on the ability of these groups to act as training instruments. The first is that, due to a lack of clear thinking about functions and consequent organisational needs, the groups are frequently ineffective at anything, including training. The second is that training has not so far emerged as a major function for the groups. Created because of feelings of isolation, they have been most successful in promoting co-operation whether in the minimal form of exchange of information or in the form of actual co-ordination on such matters as urban aid, summer play, city-wide political campaigns etc. This background has to be taken into consideration if one is going to examine the possibility that the groups might assume a training function.

THE GROUPS AND THE IDENTITY OF COMMUNITY WORK

One thing the groups have done that has a bearing on training is to help to create an identity for community work. This may seem a vague function but it has been a crucial one. The local meetings that have taken place all over the country have enabled people to see themselves as community workers, to define (although usually implicitly!) what the terms means and to convey that definition to others. It is difficult to tell, but my guess would be that the groups have played a more important role in establishing community work as a recognised field than other factors, such as the development of training facilities, literature and the efforts of ACW and CYSA. Several of them have taken this task of establishing the identity of community work further by organising meetings and conferences with councillors and local authority officials for precisely this purpose.

The attempt to educate others about the identity of community work has naturally not been a purely academic exercise. Groups that have arranged conferences, seminars and meetings on the broad issues have also acted as pressure groups for their members on issues relating to freedom of action and other conditions of work. Such issues raise basic questions about the nature of community work and it is only where groups have been fairly cohesive that they have been able to arrive at clear positions in support of members seen to be under unfair attack from their employers or others.

MORE DIRECTLY EDUCATIONAL FUNCTIONS

Because so many community workers lack formal training in their work, some local community workers' groups have assumed an educational function. But this has normally taken the form of the organisation of local seminars and conferences rather than of programmed discussion within the group itself. Moreover, it often happens that the group is not the real basis for such moves. They often come from agency-based student units or from university or polytechnic departments, while the group acts as a means of advertising the conference and as a source of speakers and resource material.

GROUP SUPERVISION AND ITS DIFFICULTIES

Although the groups have thus taken some slightly hesitant steps in the direction of self-training on general issues either of principle (e.g. community work and politics) or of technical knowledge (e.g. planning law), there has been very little development of group supervision among them. The term 'supervision' will be familiar to those community workers with knowledge of social work and some other professions[1] but might confuse others. It carries, of course, possible connotations of control and direction. But it is also used by several professions to refer to what is essentially an educational process in which the worker (or student on fieldwork placement) is encouraged and enabled to consider his work in a more critical way in the light of general principles. It is, of course, only in this educational sense that one might have expected some form of supervision to have developed within the community workers' groups. But this has not happened in spite of the fact that the groups appear to have been brought into existence partly because community workers felt the lack of the sort of support and evaluation that supervision provides in other fields of social welfare.

This might seem odd at first, but there are several good reasons for it.

Where membership of the group is fairly open there is likely to be a constant shifting of membership which makes it difficult for people to engage in the kind of serious discussion that supervision requires whether in group or one-to-one situations. An element in this is that several agencies are likely to be involved. At the very least this must restrict the area of common concern. It may also be that relations between workers, while friendly, are not so good as to make it easy for a worker to confess to failures in the presence of people from other agencies. The meetings may be too far apart to allow discussion of issues at a time when they are most crucial to the worker concerned. There is also the point that at least some of the members are likely to be receiving the support that good supervision provides within their own agencies and these are the workers most likely to appreciate the advantages of good educational supervision. This raises a further point, that many community workers are indifferent or even hostile to educational supervision because they have had little experience of it or have had particularly bad experience of it.

All these points are merely particular instances of the basic dilemma that would face any community workers' group that wished to undertake some form of educational supervision. In a useful article aimed at social workers Fizdale distinguishes 'peer supervision' and 'group supervision'.[2] In peer supervision no one assumes permanent leadership, and responsibility for the discussion of work is shared by all participants. In group supervision there is a supervisor who is necessarily in some way separate from the group. The loosely knit nature of most community workers' groups and the fact that such groups will normally be made up of people from different agencies and professional backgrounds makes peer supervision practically impossible. Only strong group cohesion will permit the informal but highly disciplined discussion that is the basis of peer supervision. But it is difficult to envisage how a supervisor could be found who was generally acceptable for the purposes of group supervision. It would also be difficult to see how the activities of that person as group supervisor would connect with the activity of the group in co-ordinating aspects of fieldwork.

POSSIBLE SOLUTIONS TO THE PROBLEM

There are some ways round the dilemma, none of them entirely satisfactory.

The group may decide to set aside some meetings at each of which the work of a particular member will be discussed. This has several advantages. It gives members a clearer idea of what their colleagues do. It allows the person subjecting his own work to discussion an opportunity to reflect with colleagues on some fundamental issues in relation to the work rather than simply as issues for debate. It thereby introduces to the group the idea of co-operative analysis of work undertaken and may serve as a basis for future discussion along such lines. It seems to me a useful proceeding as far as it goes. But obviously it does not go very far. Even if all those presenting their work do so in a serious manner and not casually or with a view to impress, it is difficult to move from that point on to a situation in which workers will normally submit difficulties, opportunities and decisions to discussion in the group.

A second approach is to have sessions on particular areas of work, perhaps with a new 'supervisor' for each session who is a regular member of the group and experienced in that particular field. Thus at one meeting one might have someone acting as group leader in a discussion on the work of members involved in General Improvement Areas and at another an entirely different person leading a discussion on the work of members involved in neighbourhood care schemes. Experience in social work suggests that this is an awkward way of organising group supervision and it has often been dropped by those who have experimented with it.[3] This is partly because it is not very flexible. It becomes difficult to raise particular problems for discussion when they arise because they do not fit in with the subject of the day. There is an additional problem with community workers' groups. Because they have a co-ordinating function they are likely to slip from discussion of the work that is being done into discussion of possible joint action. This may be a reasonable response to the raising of problems in a group supervision session. But it may also be a means of evading the uncomfortable task of discussing the effectiveness of the worker whose operations are the subject of the debate.

A third solution is to set aside some meetings of the group for group supervision and to appoint someone from outside as an educational supervisor, probably a training officer or academic from a local course. This might work very well. I do not know of anyone who had tried it. There would obviously be an initial difficulty for any group in finding someone willing to take on this work and able to do it well. (The ability to teach well academically does not automatically involve the ability to engage in fieldwork supervision well.) But, if it were possible, it would be useful. The point to notice here, however, is that this is less an instance of the group's providing itself with group supervision than of the group's acting once again as a means of locating a constituency for a particular form of training provided by an outsider.

CONCLUSION

In common with many community workers I feel that in the development of community work training far more emphasis needs to be given to training within frameworks other than that of the one or two year course than was given by the majority of those involved in producing the discussion paper published by the Central Council for Education and Training in Social Work.[4] At first glance the local community workers' groups might seem to offer a particularly useful opportunity for training outside the academic establishments. They have, indeed, enabled many community workers to develop an understanding of their role, to share experiences with colleagues and to acquire new knowledge, particularly in the form of hard information. But I believe that their role in training is necessarily a limited one. It is not merely that many of the groups suffer from a lack of clarity about their objectives and consequent defects in organisation at the moment. Insofar as the groups have clarified their objectives it has been to see themselves as means of co-ordinating field-work. This need not exclude a training function. It may even require it if effective co-ordination involves the passing on of knowledge about law or procedures or local politics to members who are inexperienced in a particular field. But the groups are such that their training role seems likely to remain a strictly subordinate one.

REFERENCES

1 On supervision as seen by social workers see, for example, Dorothy E. Pettes, *Supervision in Social Work* (London, George Allen & Unwin, 1967). On supervision in relation to community work see chapters by Bryant and Holmes and Harris in this volume.
2 Ruth Fizdale, 'Peer-group Supervision', *Social Casework*, Vol. 39, No. 8 (October 1958), pp. 443-50.
3 For example, see Donald M. Smith, 'Group Supervision: An Experience', *Social Work Today*, Vol. 3, No. 8 (13th July, 1972), pp. 13-15.
4 Central Council for Education and Training in Social Work, *The Teaching of Community Work* (CCETSW Paper 8). See especially paras 5.01-5.08.

PART II

THEORIES FOR PRACTICE

INTRODUCTION TO PART II

Community work draws for its general and practice theories upon, firstly, a variety of disciplines and fields of study, and, secondly, a large number of other and often related practices such as social work, education, planning and trade unionism. Studies like political science, social policy and social administration are incorporated into training programmes for community workers with relatively little controversy. Others are the subject of much debate and contention, and these include, for instance, many theories and concepts that community workers abstract from sociology, anthropology, philosophy and psychology, and from studies that attempt to understand and conceptualise behaviour in different types of groups.

This part of the book contains papers that deal with selected knowledge and theories that we identify as pertinent to community work. Peter Leonard stresses the importance of education and training that is based on dialogue. In particular, he suggests that 'the relationship between community workers and the social sciences should be one of dialogue and critique, rather than passive acceptance'. Leonard indicates that community workers should be aware that the way in which they draw upon, organise and use theories and models from the social sciences is influenced by their particular values and political assumptions.

Leonard mentions the contribution of research methods and theories of group behaviour in the training of community workers, and these two aspects are the subject of the chapters by John Lambert and Nano McCaughan. Lambert argues that research for a community worker cannot be a substitute for discussion and decision over matters of value and strategy, but can contribute to that debate. He suggests that community workers be critical in the ways they use research methods and findings and describes particular methods like participant observation, the use of existing sources of data and more formal methods of investigation like the social survey.

The chapter by Nano McCaughan emphasises that a group is something more than the collection of individuals who comprise it. She reviews a number of theories concerned, for example, with communication, decision making and deviance in small groups, as well as indicating the knowledge that is available about intergroup and large group behaviour. People who work with groups are often puzzled by the incidents and relationships that occur within them and which often affect the ability of the group to achieve its goals (the behaviour of the over-dominant member, for instance). McCaughan suggests that a community worker's understanding of these kinds of problems, and thus his contribution to the work of neighbourhood groups, may be enhanced by a grasp of theories relating to the behaviour and dynamics of small groups.

Community groups, community workers and other professionals have to manage their affairs, determine priorities, make decisions and plan and allocate resources. Although management in local and central government is often the target of the change efforts of community groups, the paper by Jimmy Algie, Clive Miller, and Norman Kam indicates that theories and knowledge from management and organisation studies may be useful in understanding, and better achieving, some of the above tasks.

Nicholas Derricourt suggests that 'the purpose of training is to enable workers to know what they are doing and so to be able to evaluate it'. Derricourt argues for a 'direct experience' model of training in community work that is 'firmly anchored in the concrete experience of inhabitants of working-class localities'. The chapter is a helpful link with the final part of the book to the extent that Derricourt emphasises the value of linking the teaching of theory to the field experience of community work students.

It is difficult to assess the usefulness to practitioners of material from other disciplines for it is often found in a form that is not readily usable in practice. Rothman, for instance, has indicated the issues and difficulties in deriving practice principles for community workers from research in the social sciences.[1] Despite the complex nature of deriving utility from the interaction of theory and practice, it remains an important requirement of the ideas, theories and knowledge (including those reviewed in the following chapters) upon which community work often draws, that they can be developed by workers to help them better to understand phenomena encountered in their practice, and thus better to work with community groups towards the achievement of their goals. It may be an equally desirable and necessary requirement of community workers that they are able, as Peter Leonard argues in his chapter, to analyse their practice and 'to contribute to the development of middle range explanatory theories about community "problems" and community action so that [their] practice can rest upon firmer foundations'.

REFERENCE

1 Jack Rothman, *Planning and Organising for Social Change* (Columbia University Press, 1974). On the translation of theory into practice, see chapter 11.

Chapter 5

THE CONTRIBUTION OF THE SOCIAL SCIENCES: IDEOLOGY AND EXPLANATION

Peter Leonard

INTRODUCTION

It is appropriate to begin the examination of the contribution of the social sciences to community work from a stance of considerable scepticism. Doubts about the value of the social sciences for community work must stem from two interrelated sources. Firstly, there is the question of the professional purposes of drawing on the social sciences. In a growing occupation like community work, some sections of which aspire to professional status, the development of a manifest social science base is a prerequisite for success. Once the training of community workers is firmly wedded to the existing educational institutions, a corresponding apparatus of study must be established as a means of academic legitimation and a justification for the employment of a range of social science teaching and research staff – sociologists, economists, social psychologists, and others. Alongside the status, power and rewards which come to occupations that can claim a 'scientific' base, there are other consequences of the impact of the social sciences: the mystification and social distancing which appears to accompany professionalisation.

Secondly, important as these points of reservation may be, of more profound significance is the problem of the function of the social sciences generally within society. Briefly, the social sciences may be seen as the intellectual and ideological products of a particular kind of social order. The function of these disciplines may then be to provide legitimation for existing economic and political structures, by both *explaining* them and, through various forms of application, providing intellectual and 'scientific' support for a range of social policies, including the development of community work, which will preserve intact the main features of the social order. It may be argued that such preservation does not coincide with the material interests of the people with whom community workers are primarily engaged in various forms of action.

These are serious objections to the utilisation of the social sciences in community work and will be explored in various contexts as this chapter proceeds. At this stage, however, we should make the following points: first, that the social sciences have a more contradictory, ambiguous relationship to the existing social structures than the foregoing argument might suggest; but, second, that because we must recognise the social and political function of the social sciences we should be prepared to explore various philosophical and sociological perspectives on knowledge if we are to take an active, critical stance. The most dangerous and politically naive approach to social sciences utilisation is that which concentrates exclusively on narrowly defined problems of the practical application of social science theories and ignores the more fundamental issues involved. In what follows, then, we shall attempt to identify and explore a number of questions surrounding the relationship of the social sciences to community work, firstly examining some of the philosophical and theoretical problems involved, and secondly by looking at how the practice and context of community work suggest the utilisation of specific areas of knowledge.

In writing this chapter, I have been faced with a basic problem of exposition: should we begin with theory and then move to practice, or should we start with the problems of practice and then relate them to social science theories? I have already suggested why I think that some theoretical issues should be tackled first, but such a starting-point might be taken to signify the superiority of theory over practice, of *ideas* over the material reality which community workers are struggling with. As I do not believe this to be the case, I have clearly not been able to avoid confronting a problem which is central to the issues we are concerned with: the relation of knowledge to the material world and to our activities within it. It is therefore important that we begin our main theoretical discussions by focus on this issue.

TWO TYPES OF THEORY

Our starting-point in looking at the relationship between theory and practice (for example, does theory emerge from practice or does practice emerge from theory?) is to distinguish broadly between the two kinds of theory that community workers are concerned with.

The first type of theory we might denote as *descriptive and explanatory*. We meet this type of theory as the typical product of the social sciences. The social scientist's analysis of events includes an account of how something happened and why it happened. Thus we are provided with explanation of the effects of maternal deprivation or poverty, of the consequences of the development of large-scale organisations, or of the relationship between various types of industrial development and the structure of communities. The importance of this type of theory lies in its attempt to identify causal relationships between events:

'If we are not shown how one part of a social process is causally related to another part, of how one aspect of an activity is causally connected to another, we are given no analysis of either an activity or a process.'[1]

Community workers certainly look to social science theories to provide explanations of *causes*. But these explanations are not, for the community worker, an end in themselves, but are seen as contributing to the development of the second type of theory, which is *prescriptive*. Prescriptive theory attempts to outline principles and strategies of action within particular contexts. Thus, on the basis of descriptive and explanatory theory from the social sciences and other sources, various policies and practices are developed to attempt to prevent maternal deprivation or poverty, or to mitigate its effects; strategies are invented to combat the effects of large-scale organisations; and community activists learn the means by which to resist the cultural elimination involved in much of urban planning.

Obviously, this latter type of theory is substantially different from the former type: it is a theory of practice rather than a theory of explanation, although it incorporates explanatory theory within it. Community work theory is a particular example of an attempt to develop a practice theory. Clearly, unlike social science theory, it is not an autonomous form of knowledge, or an autonomous discipline. Because it is concerned with what *ought* to be done in a range of practical activities many of its central operations are, in fact, moral and political questions of a particular level of generality.

The distinction we have made between the two types of theory might lead us to assume that while prescriptive theory is concerned with moral and political issues, explanatory theory in the social sciences is value-free. However, this is not an assumption which can easily be made and it leads us to the next stage in our discussion: the different perspectives that exist on the nature of the social sciences themselves.

MODELS OF SOCIAL SCIENCE

In a recently published paper[2] I have elaborated a framework within which to examine the different perspectives on the social sciences, Here, I shall cover the ground briefly in a way which will, I hope, provide some guide to community workers when they confront some of the claims of the social sciences to provide relevant and usable knowledge. Controversy about the success or failure of the social sciences to provide adequate explanations of social phenomena usually centres on two different and opposite kinds of argument. On the one side, it is suggested that the social sciences should be seen as parallel to the physical sciences, should provide similar kinds of explanations and will be able to in the long run. Alternatively, it is argued that the social sciences do not and ought not resemble the physical sciences and that therefore the explanations that they provide are of a quite different kind.

Thus we have basically two different models of the social sciences, one which we can call a *physical sciences model* and the other a *human sciences model*. The former model demands social science aspiration to physical sciences methodology, with measurement and objectivity as an essential component. It argues that careful empirical study of observable data, tested against well formulated hypotheses, is the essential prerequisite of scientific activity. Within this model, behaviourist psychology,[3] certain types of empirical sociology, and econometrics are clear examples, whilst, as Karl Popper[4] and Peter Medawar[5] have argued, Marxism and psychoanalysis are but two areas of knowledge which could not be considered to be scientific. If the 'proper' social sciences are able to achieve a similar degree of rigour to that of the physical sciences, then, the argument runs, it is possible for them to be value-free and thus provide objective knowledge on which to base social policies.

The conflicting, human sciences model starts from the contention either that there is a basic discontinuity between the study of social as compared with physical phenomena, or, more usually, that even the physical sciences are not as objective and value-free as is often argued. In any case, protagonists within this model generally maintain that subjective understanding is an essential part of the social scientists' approach to his phenomena of study and that because of the identification of the scientist with his material, values are bound to enter into his activity. Thus the kinds of sociology most influenced by Weber, the recent deviancy theory drawing upon phenomenology and ethnomethodology[6] and psychoanalytic theory are all examples of social science activity within the human sciences model. Within this model, however, we must also place those who emphasise the importance of locating the social sciences firmly within an analysis of society and its social institutions. This is the focus of the seminal work of a number of the sociologists of knowledge.[7] A specific example of this approach is also to be seen in the work of Marxist philosophers[8] who maintain that we must see the social sciences of capitalism as products in part of an oppressive social structure based on class exploitation. What such a perspective suggests is that in drawing upon the theories and data of the social sciences full attention should be given to their explicit or hidden ideological foundations and assumptions.[9]

In utilising social science theories, then, community workers need to evaluate them in terms of what overall view of the social sciences they are based upon. By this means we are able to know what is counted as evidence to support a theory, and how it purports to relate to moral and political issues. Although we can draw successfully on some theories and data developed within a physical sciences model, the perspective of this chapter is firmly within the human sciences model in general and the Marxist perspective in particular. Thus I am arguing that community workers need some understanding of the sociology of knowledge, including the origins, ideological basis and connection with class and other interests of any particular contribution from the social sciences, as well as its practical relevance to action.

KNOWLEDGE AND THE MATERIAL WORLD

Whilst such a stance in relation to the social sciences is certainly a critical one, it is important, if we are to utilise the social sciences effectively, that we recognise the *complexity* of the relationship between the social sciences and the social structure. If we do not, we may be led to ignore the positive contributions which the social sciences can make even though they reflect, in part, an oppressive social structure. In order to clarify this point, we need to make a philosophical detour in order to examine the relationship between ideas and the material world. The understanding we might gain from this examination will help us, as we shall see later, in working out the nature of the *relationship* that community workers should develop with the social sciences.

The question we are now to try to answer is this: what is the relationship between our understanding of the world (our ideas, our consciousness) and the material world itself? One answer to the question we might term *vulgar materialism*, where consciousness is seen as entirely determined by the material (and social) world. Thus some behaviourist psychologists would see human behaviour, including ideas, as ultimately determined by genetic and environmental factors. Similarly, some approaches to socialisation see it as eventually a one-way process in which the culture imprints the human being with his ideas and values. In such a highly mechanistic conception of man, our relationship to knowledge is a very restricted one. Its genesis is entirely dependent on material conditions, and such a view tends to encourage a fatalistic relationship to knowledge as a *given*, as relatively unproblematic. In contrast is the *idealist* position, in which ideas and consciousness generally are independent variables or even determine the man-made material world. Knowledge is essentially independent of the social structure, and social science theories are a 'free creation of the human intellect'.[10] One view is that human knowledge is basically about subjective understanding and man is quite 'free of the world' in the creation of his ideas.[11] The most important implication of this position is that argued by Barry Hindess in his critique of the phenomenological and ethnomethodological approach to deviance, namely that it denies the *possibility* of knowing the external world. He suggests that this position leads 'inexorably to the denial of the possibility of rational knowledge, that this denial cannot be restricted to a limited domain of the materials used by sociologists, and that it must apply in full generality to all forms of rational knowledge'.[12]

The problems we encounter in both vulgar materialist and idealist views on knowledge lead us to argue for more complex answers to the question of the relationship between human consciousness and the material world. This view, *dialectical materialism*, suggests that consciousness and the material world interact upon each other.[13] Whilst the material world, particularly the modes of economic production and the resulting social structure, have a predominant influence in their interaction, human consciousness is important in determining how the possibilities of the material world shall be used. Because knowledge, understanding and consciousness are not straight reflections of the material world, *false consciousness* is, to a degree, the experience of all human beings. Such a view of knowledge, whilst it alerts us to the relationship between the social sciences and the social structure, maintains that the one is not simply a mirror reflection of the other, but that ideas can be generated which are contradictory to the social structure and which themselves can contribute to social change.

CRITICAL APPROACHES TO KNOWLEDGE

The purpose of this philosophical detour has been to lay some foundations for the argument that the relationship between community workers and the social sciences should be one of dialogue and critique rather than passive acceptance. In creating such a relationship with social science knowledge, however, we are faced with substantial obstacles. The predominant model of education which we experience and which may strongly influence our attitude to the social sciences, we may refer to as *cultural transmission*. Education is conceived of substantially as a mechanistic socialisation process in which 'valuable' knowledge is transmitted from teacher to student.[14] Although progressive education has attempted to develop alternative models, nevertheless the cultural transmission model exercises a predominant influence in education, including professional education. Paulo Freire[15] has argued that this 'banking' model operates on the principle that knowledge is to be deposited in people who are empty vessels to be filled. Such an approach to education, he maintains, reflects an oppressive social system and the requirements of ruling-class interests. He proposes a liberating approach to knowledge which is based on dialogue intended to raise the critical consciousness of all those involved in the process, a consciousness which combats fatalism and challenges the established social order.

The relationship of community workers to the social sciences should, I am maintaining, be of a dialogical kind. The connection between the social sciences and the social structure must be understood critically and its ideological foundations explored. In particular, the over-deterministic stance of social science theories which, when added together, give an unremitting picture of men and women as totally determined by genetic, intra-psychic and environmental circumstances, should be resisted. Such determinism allows little opportunity for radical change and reinforces the fatalism which a passive relationship to the social sciences involves.

So far in this chapter we have approached the problem of the contribution of the social sciences to community work by examining a number of theoretical and philosophical issues. We have tackled our problem from a primarily deductive standpoint, moving from overall theoretical concepts as a basis for the examination of specific issues of practice. But this is only one part in the process of the development of knowledge. I shall argue that inductive approaches, where the practitioner, on the basis of his practice experience, contributes to the development of theory, are equally important. Such theory development from the field has two effects: it ensures that existing social science theory is critically tested in a way which highlights the extent to which it fails to explain the phenomena with which the practitioner is working, and it also adds new knowledge to the social sciences themselves. The process of knowledge development, then, must be seen as a dialectic between deductive and inductive approaches, a continuous interaction between theory and practice. The fusing of theory and practice, where understanding the work and changing it are part of the same process, should be a major objective of community work itself.

Given the overall critical stance in relation to the social sciences that I have outlined, how does the community worker more specifically relate social science theory to his practice? The general orientation of this paper would not be expected to lead to highly specific recommendations, or to detailed bibliographies. We can, however, suggest the *method* by which community workers can approach the social sciences. I shall suggest two stages: first, identifying the alternative overall models of community problems, and second, formulating a framework within which community work practice can be located.

GENERAL THEORETICAL MODELS

In exploring the different models of community problems, we are faced immediately both with the great range of definitions of community which sociologists have developed, and, more importantly, with the multitude of ideological purposes behind the whole concept of community.[16] In the current debate about the nature and causes of community problems and the objectives of social policy responses, we are able in very broad terms to distinguish between *social disorganisation* and *structural conflict* models.[17]

The *social disorganisation model* has its theoretical roots in much of the mainstream literature of economics, sociology, social administration, political science and psychology.[18] It is based upon the assumption that in Western societies the state represents, albeit imperfectly, the interests of the whole population through a democratic political process. However, these societies face a series of problems in attempting to ensure that all of the population benefits from industrial and social development. For some social scientists, individual, family or community pathology is the major problem to be tackled. Community problems of deviance, including lack of effective socialisation to the dominant cultural norms, arise from the internal pathology of the poor. This pathology is often transmitted from generation to generation. Clearly a good deal of the work on the culture of poverty, on maternal deprivation, and on the cycle of deprivation is important within this model. The social policy response is primarily therapeutic and compensatory. Alongside this focus on the poor and deprived there is also developing a view of community problems which takes account of the failure of organisations themselves. Particularly important here is the range of work being undertaken on the relationship between the school and the community and on the problems and failures of urban planning. Studies of bureaucracy and especially those which explore the interaction between welfare organisations and their consumers are also relevant here. In general, approaches within this model, and it is the dominant one, view the Welfare State as primarily benign and the problems which arise within it as defects which can be overcome given the more appropriate use of resources within the existing economic and political structure.

The *structural conflict model* has very different theoretical roots as the basis of an alternative analysis of community problems and social policy responses. It is primarily based on a Marxist theory of the state and of the social system under capitalism.[19] Fundamental to this model is a view of the Welfare State as an expression, in part, of ruling-class interests and of community problems being reflections of more profound issues stemming from the imperatives of capitalist modes of production. It is argued that the deprivation, poverty and disadvantage which is experienced by many of the neighbourhoods in which community work takes place are direct results of the effects of the economy on the working class in general and the unskilled sections of it in particular. The Welfare State, and often community work within it, functions primarily in order to ameliorate, homogenise and, if possible, culturally eliminate lower working-class neighbourhoods that might provide a source of deviant politics. Within this model, the emphasis of social science study is on the class structure and its effects, the ways in which central and local government reflect sectional interests, and the development of a political economy of the Welfare State which includes an analysis of the social services as a means for the reproduction of labour.[20] The community work response of those who broadly accept this model will focus on strategies for the redistribution of power and control through the development of the political consciousness of working-class communities.[21]

Obviously, this is a very simplistic analysis of the different models of community problems and policy responses; its purpose, however, is merely to indicate that the selection of social science materials for community work is likely to be strongly influenced by the ideological stance of the community worker. The overarching theory of the state and of society which the community worker develops needs to be made explicit; he can then approach the more specific empirical literature within both models with a critical apparatus capable of evaluating it.

PRACTICE AND THE SOCIAL SCIENCES

Whilst this first stage in the process of orientation to the social sciences provides the community worker with some general guidelines, he also needs a means of selecting social science contributions which relate directly to the *process* of community work. In this second stage he will map out a practice framework which both locates the worker in relation to relevant others and identifies the major elements in the process of community work intervention itself. It is not within the scope of this paper to suggest such a framework in detail; we can, however, indicate in general terms some of the elements in the framework and a few examples of the social science contributions that are relevant to them.

There are four quite obvious elements in a practice framework which we can identify immediately: the community or neighbourhood in whose interest community work is ostensibly undertaken; the local organisational and political context; the wider structural variables; the community work intervention process itself.

The approach to the idea of *community and neighbourhood* should, we have suggested, begin with an exploration of its sociological significance and ideological roots.[22] Beyond this a wide range of social science literature becomes relevant. Of particular interest are sociological and anthropological studies of small community and neighbourhood cultures,[23] including immigrant cultures and their relationship to the host community. An understanding of the economic and social history of an area is of substantial importance to the community worker, for it provides a perspective within which to place the present cultural patterns.[24] In this context also, studies of working-class politics are of importance.[25]

In understanding the *local organisational and political context* of community work, the study of local government and the particular features of the local political party organisation is essential,[26] for community workers sometimes fail to analyse effectively the relationship between, for example, the party caucus, the local councillor and the ward which he represents. The study of bureaucracy is also clearly essential here, though once again it is important to explore carefully the ideological assumptions which underlie the various approaches to organisational analysis.[27]

Some of the *wider structural variables* within which community work takes place were identified when we looked at the alternative models of the state and of society. Obviously these variables include the study of the major social institutions, such as education and production. In this context also comes the study of the family as a social institution; the recent literature which elaborates a critical analysis of the family from women's standpoint is particularly important.[28]

Another element in the practice framework which will guide the community worker in his selection of social science material is the *process of community work intervention*. Here he will be able to draw, firstly, on the literature which helps him with the task of defining the problems with which he will work. Problem definition cannot, as we have seen, be taken for granted but must be understood as socially constructed; here the sociological work on deviance and labelling processes will be of value.[29] Secondly, the community worker is involved in a range of data collection activities. Whilst he may draw on the standard literature on research methods in the social sciences, it will be important also to take full account of the critical work on methodology which is producing a reaction against the more traditional kinds of empirical research.[30] Thirdly, in his negotiations and interaction with neighbourhood groups, staff groups and other collectivities, he will be able to draw on a vast range of work on group behaviour from the fields of social psychology and sociology.[31] In his work with groups he may be engaged in drawing on social science literature in his educational functions, in developing strategies for policy and organisational change, in welfare rights activism and in building an organisation himself.

In many of the activities merely sketched in here, the community workers will, however, be operating at the frontiers of social science knowledge or beyond them. The contribution of the social sciences is often such that the theories available are too crude and imperfect to account for the complexities of practice. It is because of this that we have suggested, in this latter section, that the community worker should attempt to conceptualise his practice within a framework which enables him to draw critically on what the social sciences have to offer. In addition, however, he will need to contribute to the development of middle-range explanatory theories about community problems and community action so that his practice can rest upon firmer foundations.

CONCLUSION

In this chapter, we have argued that a critical, even sceptical stance in relation to the social sciences is the appropriate one. It has been suggested that the community worker should both take account of some of the major philosophical and ideological issues involved and also identify his own model of problems and practice if he is to utilise the social sciences effectively. In proposing that community workers should work from the basis of a systematic overall theoretical perspective which provides an account of the state and a general explanation of social problems, are we limiting ourselves to a rigid framework and neglecting the advantages that can come from a pragmatic eclecticism? Eclecticism, as the history of much of social administration and criminology has shown, is a mixed blessing. The lack of an overall theoretical perspective within which empirical data and practice experience can be located can lead to fragmentation and to a failure to analyse critically the common-sense definitions of institutions and problems which bombard us daily and which saturate the dominant culture. Because community work is concerned centrally with moral and political issues, we are well advised to clarify our ideological assumptions and relate these to the major social science theories.

Although we must identify the overarching theory which lies at the base of our perspectives on the state and society, this does not mean that the theory must be impervious to change. If the overall theoretical perspective fails to account for the empirical data we encounter in our practice experience, a number of alternatives are available to us. We may abandon the theory completely, we may try to ignore the contrary evidence, or we may attempt to modify the theory to take account of the new evidence. Whilst ignoring the evidence which appears to refute some part of our theoretical basis is always mistaken, we are not necessarily obliged to move to the extreme of dramatic abandonment of the theory. Revisionism has an important place in theoretical development.

REFERENCES

1 R. Brown, *Explanation in Social Science* (London, Routledge & Kegan Paul, 1963), p. 24.
2 P. Leonard, 'Explanation and Education in Social Work', *British Journal of Social Work*, vol. 5, No. 3 (1975).
3 See B. F. Skinner, *Beyond Freedom and Dignity* (London, Penguin Books, 1973).
4 K. R. Popper, *The Poverty of Historicism* (London, Routledge & Kegan Paul, 1960). For an alternative view read G. Lichtheim, *Marxism* (London, Routledge & Kegan Paul, 1961).
5 P. B. Medawar, *Induction and Intuition in Scientific Thought* (London, Methuen, 1969).
6 For a general review which includes this perspective see I. Taylor, P. Walton and J. Young, *The New Criminology* (London, Routledge & Kegan Paul, 1973).
7 One of the most important works in this field is P. Berger and T. Luckmann, *The Social Construction of Reality* (London, Allen Lane The Penguin Press, 1967).

8 See L. Goldmann, *The Human Sciences and Philosophy* (London, Jonathan Cape, 1969).
9 For an introduction, see R. Blackburn (ed.), *Ideology in Social Science* (London, Fontana, 1972).
10 R. C. Sheldon, 'Some Observations on Theory in the Social Sciences' in T. Parsons and E. Shils (eds), *Toward a General Theory of Action* (New York, Harper 1962), p. 31.
11 See A. Schutz, *The Phenomenology of the Social World* (London, Heinemann, 1972).
12 B. Hindess, *The Use of Official Statistics in Sociology* (London, Macmillan, 1973).
13 As an introduction see M. Cornforth, *Dialectical Materialism*, vol. 3 (London, Lawrence and Wishart, 1963). A more advanced exposition is in H. Lefebre, *Dialectical Materialism* (London, Jonathan Cape, 1968).
14 R. S. Peters, *Ethics and Education* (London, George Allen & Unwin, 1966).
15 P. Freire, *Pedagogy of the Oppressed* (London, Penguin Books, 1972).
16 See R. Plant, *Community and Ideology* (London, Routledge & Kegan Paul, 1974).
17 For the linking of community work practice to overall models, see Coventry Community Development Project, *Final Report* (March 1975), obtainable from CDP Information and Intelligence Unit, Mary Ward House, 5 Tavistock Place, London WC1H 9SS.
18 See, for example, T. Parsons, *The Social System* (London, Routledge & Kegan Paul, 1964); J. K. Galbraith, *The Affluent Society* (London, Penguin Books, 1962); and T. H. Marshall, *Social Policy*, 4th edn (London, Hutchinson, 1975). An excellent introduction to the relation of social policy to sociology is R. Pinker, *Social Theory and Social Policy* (London, Heinemann, 1971).
19 See R. Miliband, *The State in Capitalist Society* (London, Quartet Books, 1973) and articles by Edward Nell and Robin Blackburn in R. Blackburn, *Ideology in Social Science* (London, Fontana, 1972).
20 See V. George, *Social Security and Society* (London, Routledge & Kegan Paul, 1973) and D. Wedderburn, *Poverty, Inequality and the Class Structure* (Cambridge University Press, 1974).
21 As a brief introduction to the Marxist study of consciousness see M. A. Coulson and D. S. Riddell, *Approaching Sociology* (London, Routledge & Kegan Paul, 1970), ch. 5. The most important work remains G. Lukács, *History and Class Consciousness* (London, Merlin Press, 1971).
22 See Plant, op. cit. ch. 3, and C. Bell and H. Newby, *Community Studies* (London, George Allen & Unwin, 1972).
23 From the great range available, an important study remains that of J. Klein, *Samples from English Cultures* (London, Routledge & Kegan Paul, 1965), 2 vols.
24 For London, for example, see G. Stedman Jones, *Outcast London* (London, Oxford University Press, 1971).
25 See B. Hindess, *The Decline of Working Class Politics* (London, MacGibbon and Kee, 1971).
26 As one example, see W. Hampton, *Democracy and Community: A Study of Politics in Sheffield* (London, Oxford University Press, 1970).

27 There is a substantial sociological literature here, but a useful introduction is A. Etzioni, *Modern Organizations* (New Jersey, Prentice Hall, 1964). From a different standpoint see A. Gouldner, 'The Secrets of Organizations' in R. Kramer and H. Specht (eds), *Readings in Community Organization Practice* (New Jersey, Prentice Hall, 1969).
28 See S. Rowbotham, *Woman's Consciousness, Man's World* (London, Penguin Books, 1973).
29 A particularly striking example is A. V. Cicourel, *The Social Organization of Juvenile Justice* (New York, John Wiley, 1968).
30 See D. L. Phillips, *Knowledge From What?* (Chicago, Rand McNally, 1971) and A. V. Cicourel, *Cognitive Sociology* (London, Penguin Books, 1973).
31 A useful introduction is T. Mills, *The Sociology of Small Groups* (New Jersey, Prentice Hall, 1967) while the collection of studies in D. Cartwright and A. Zander (eds), *Group Dynamics* (Evanston, Row Peterson, 1960) remains an important source of reference.

Chapter 6

GROUP BEHAVIOUR: SOME THEORIES FOR PRACTICE

Nano McCaughan

Community workers are engaged for much of their time with groups – with groups of residents in the neighbourhood, as participants in discussions with service agencies and departments, or as members of staff groups in the community work project or area team. This chapter reviews some theories of group behaviour that community workers may find helpful in understanding the groups in which they work. It is divided into three parts, dealing with small group, intergroup and large group behaviour.

PART ONE: BEHAVIOUR IN SMALL GROUPS

Knowledge resulting from intuitive speculation and empirical experiments about small group behaviour that is useful to community workers has been contributed from several disciplines – sociology, social psychology, psychotherapy and anthropology. It is not possible to organise this knowledge into any one coherent model, and its usefulness must depend to a large extent on the assumptions that particular workers hold about the nature of man and society, and their own personal experiences of groups.

The definition of a small group used in this paper is that of Cartwright and Zander,[1] who defined it as a collection of people who have face-to-face interaction; the group is small enough for everyone to be known and absences noted. The purpose of the formation of the group is such that interdependence is necessary to achieve the goal, and the behaviour of one individual affects others. The members define themselves as belonging, and are usually defined so by other individuals or groups. They share time and space to meet and normally all share a model object, whether it be a leader, an activity or an ideal, through which the members can identify with one another. These properties are of sufficient generality to include such different entities as a tenants' association, a delinquent gang or some elderly people wishing to create a senior citizens' club.

TYPES OF SMALL GROUPS

There are, broadly speaking, three types of groups, and community workers will probably work with all of them.

Firstly, *groups of spontaneous formation*. Examples are a family, a street gang, a friendship peer group. Most of these groups are reference groups, and they tend to arise out of physical proximity and often have shifting boundaries. They demand less specialisation in role and more time and flexibility than specially formed groups. The influence of these groups stems from the opportunity they afford their members to satisfy a wide variety of needs. The family remains the primary model of group life in this society and merits intensive study by community workers, particularly those aspects of family interaction pertaining to cultural transmission, socialisation and control; see Bott,[2] Vogel and Bell,[3] G. Coyle,[4] M. Phillips.[5]

Secondly, there are those groups *deliberately formed for a more specific purpose*. Common examples are work groups, committees, working parties, social action groups and self-help groups. These groups come together for a limited time on the assumption that the particular problem they are trying to solve, or task they are endeavouring to complete, can be best served by pooling the resources of energy, intelligence and skill of several people.

These groups are generally referred to as task-oriented groups and have been extensively studied. An important finding has been that most effective task groups spend considerable time maintaining good personal relations in the group.[6] But if membership itself becomes too attractive and necessary, the individual's primary purpose will be to ensure the survival of the group in its present form, regardless of the demands of the work, or the external environment. Many community workers will have encountered this phenomenon in situations where residents seek to perpetuate a neighbourhood group after the attainment of its goals.

The third type of group is formed through *external designation*[7] or involuntary group membership. Individuals are designated membership of a group by others because of some common social characteristic. We will only be concerned with groups who have accepted that commonality, and been influenced by the designation. Examples are usually quite large groups: inmates of a prison or mental hospital ward, immigrants, Jews, etc. However, in a community work setting it is possible to find smaller groups of this kind: 'the squatters at No. 7', or the 'tenants of B block'.

INDIVIDUAL AND GROUP MEMBERSHIP

What motivates individuals to become members of groups involved in issues of community change? Maslow's[8] hierarchical categorisation of human needs may prove useful. He postulated five levels of needs, and indicated that if these needs at the various levels are *not* satisfied they remain as a very strong influence on motivation. At the lowest level, but pre-eminent in importance, are the *needs for physical survival*. The rewards for group action in pursuit of gratification of these needs must be extrinsic and concrete, or the individual will abandon collective action.

On the second level are the *safety needs* – the wish for protection against danger, threat and deprivation. In modern society these needs will be particularly felt if the individual feels himself to be the object of arbitrary authority, or in a dependent relationship. He is likely to find gratification in a collectivity, whose norm is interdependence and whose goal is to ensure the rights of the powerless and underprivileged.

On the next hierarchical level are *social needs*: the wish for belonging, for association with and acceptance by one's fellows, for giving and receiving friendship and love.

Above the social needs are the *ego needs*, for the affirmation of the individual's identity and value. These are of two kinds: firstly, those that relate to self-esteem, self-confidence in mastery of the environment, giving independence and a sense of achievement and competence; and, secondly, needs that relate to one's reputation in the eyes of others – the need for status among peers, for recognition, appreciation and deserved respect.

Finally, at the highest level are the *needs for self-fulfilment*: the drive towards realising one's fullest potential, to continue one's self-development, to become creative (in the widest sense). The first three levels of needs broadly correspond with the product goals of community work, and the ego and self-fulfilment needs with its process goals.

We live in a society which has created institutions to ensure the fulfilment of first and second level needs – the welfare state, the police, trade unions, etc. But the community worker will frequently discover individuals who are deprived in these areas, particularly in times or regions of high unemployment, with large families, and inadequate housing. If the professional has not himself experienced this deprivation it will be difficult for him to understand the strength of feeling and anxiety attached to the motivation to fulfil those individual needs, sometimes at the expense of other members in the neighbourhood group.

Many people in this industrialised and urban environment have insufficient opportunity to explore means for fulfilling the higher level needs. If they have been consistently frustrated in school, in the local community, at work, individuals may manifest indolence, passivity and resistance to efforts made to bring about change. Maslow suggests that man is largely self-motivating; it is difficult to motivate him except in so far as one can attempt to get him to achieve his own goals by directing efforts to the group goals. Most adults involved in community life are motivated by a mixture of self-interest and interest devoted to the group cause. The tasks and interactional structure of any group must take account of this admixture and adapt to the best possible balance.

THE INTERACTIVE PROCESS IN A GROUP

1 Group Goals

In a newly formed group the first task is the selection of a goal or outcome that is congruant both with the purposes of individual members and with the intention of the initiators of the group. We have discussed person-oriented motives for group membership. In community work activities the groups are usually intended to serve group-oriented motives, or outcomes favourable to the group and a wider constituency. Cartwright and Zander[9] discuss three aspects of goal-seeking behaviour: (a) the identification of the group's goal (this is often a general goal which is difficult to operationalise, e.g. 'to improve housing facilities for immigrants in a neighbourhood'); (b) the location of the group in relation to the goal; and (c) the identification of action to be undertaken to move the group closer to its goal.

An important study for community workers is that of Raven and Reitsema[10] which throws some light on the relationship between clarity of goal and the paths to achieve it, and on the interpersonal relations in the group. Clarity of goal was found to increase the attractiveness of the group, to increase task-related activities, reduce hostile feelings to other members and give a greater sense of belonging to the individual, who rated both his own performance and that of the group more highly when the goal was clear.

2 Role Structure in Groups

Although groups may have periods when their activities appear to lack structure, studies indicate that the members rapidly form structures in their interpersonal relations. This appears to stem from the needs of individuals to experience predictability in others and to form some stability in their relations. One can generally find two kinds of structural relations in a group – formal (related to task activities) and informal (related to interpersonal attraction and similarity). The demands of the latter can be as potent and influential as the former. See Whyte[11] and Homans.[12]

The technique of sociometry was introduced by Moreno[13] in 1934 as a device useful for assessing interpersonal attraction, rejection and (implicitly) power. By observation of the amount of time spent together, verbal and non-verbal communication, physical proximity, as well as by asking members who they would choose to associate with in undertaking different tasks, or in different social situations, a picture can be built up of the alliances in a group. Sociometric charts reveal isolates, pairs, small subgroups, rivalries and competitive alliances. From the application of sociometry in research studies[14] we find that effective groups like each other more as individuals, and that group members involved in a difficult and frustrating task will tend to dislike each other more and disintegrate. Detailed knowledge of the affective structure of a group can be used by community workers to enhance its functioning. If members are attracted to one another they will work more cohesively together on a task that must be performed quickly; and one can determine whose leadership would be most acceptable for a particular activity.

Small groups have always problems to solve in achieving a balance between two sets of demands. Firstly, there are the demands of goal achievement and adaptation to external pressures and opportunities. These require leadership to initiate action, risk and change. Secondly, there are the demands for internal integration and resolution of emotional tensions in the service of group cohesiveness and survival. Individuals, unless they are extremely gifted and flexible, will run into trouble if they try to meet both demands at the same time. Part of the autonomy one has to give up in joining a group is reflected in this conflict; the 'ideas' man must suffer a certain amount of dislike and distance, the popular and sympathetic 'group maintainer' must repress ideas and disagreement, to his inner discomfort.

In a seminal study about rôle differentiation in small problem-solving groups Bales[15] found some consistent and common roles. Performance was scored on activity, task ability and likeability ratings:

the member who ranks high on all three, who corresponds to the stereotype of the 'good leader' or 'great man'. Rarely found;
the member who scores high on activity and task but low on likeability, deemed the 'task specialist'. Commonly found and often works co-operatively with the next category;
the member who is high on likeability but low on the other criteria, deemed the 'social specialist';
the member who is high on activity and low on the other two, whom Bales called the 'over-active deviant'. Shows domination rather than leadership;
the member who scores low on all three, called 'under-active' deviant; may be a kind of scapegoat.

In other studies[16] it has been found that many groups operate under a dual leadership of task and social specialists. The task-centred leader tends to be progressively disliked and must rely on the co-operation of the socio-emotional leader, whose actions are geared to reduce hostility and tension, enhance members' self-evaluation, and look after the physical and psychological comfort of the members. The community worker may often function quite actively as a socio-emotional leader in groups, and this function has been described by Thomas.[17]

(3) *Communication in Groups*
Groups are dependent on an effective communication system, both in working on their internal agendas and in their interactions with individuals and other groups in their environment. Three aspects of communication will be of importance to the community worker: body language, language codes and verbal transactions, and patterns of communication structure.

Body Language. Body language can either confuse, contradict or interfere with the message being transmitted in speech.[18] Complex non-verbal cues are given and received on an information level to indicate social position, attitudes to the relative position of the other, and emotion or lack of it relevant to present interaction. Additionally, Alinsky has commented on how information about the values and life style of community workers is communicated through their dress, hairstyle, mannerisms, language and accent.[19] The writer has noted in groups that a silent member, or one whose stance indicates boredom or disgust with the proceedings, can have a substantial influence on the group's interaction and will often be reacted to as a deviant member.

Language Codes and Verbal Transactions. When we talk we transmit a message which is weighed up by others in the light of many variables and responded to when an assessment has been made. What is taken into account are accent and grammar and body language in new interactions; the history of previous messages, congruence between words and effect of delivery, and what one wishes to hear in familiar interactions.

The work of Basil Bernstein[20] on language codes is of relevance to all social and community workers. He labelled as 'codes' speech which differed in its function: that with a strong social function he called 'restricted' and that with the function of communicating and developing ideas and plans he called 'elaborate'. Bernstein contended that these codes were used differently in middle- and working-class cultures: that middle-class people were able to use both appropriately, but many working-class people had access only to a restricted code because of educational and family socialisation processes. Thomas has provided an interesting example of the different responses to advice giving and taking of working-class residents and middle-class play leaders.[21]

Patterns of Communication. The third aspect of communication covers patterns of communication networks and their effect on group behaviour. In free communication situations equal participation is not usual, and groups appear to adopt spontaneously a gradient of activity rates among the members. Members who talk most receive most interactions, and this pattern quickly stabilises.[22] In structured groups, members with high status, particularly in the task area, give and receive most communications. High status members tend to communicate more to each other; low status members communicate more to high status members, often in terms of giving feedback rather than initiating new ideas or suggestions. Bavelas[23] has developed some different communication patterns from observations of various groups both within organisations and outside. His findings may be of considerable use in helping community workers understand, for instance, the effect of different seating arrangements in groups on the way people communicate with one another.

(4) Decision Making in Groups

This important topic has been generously studied by small group theorists, and we will consider four aspects that need to be considered when one is involved in group decision making.

Process. Bales and Strodtbeck[24] have outlined a logical and tested sequence of events which occur under certain common conditions. The conditions take into account the problem to be solved, and the group composition (size, variety of membership, etc.). They found that most groups move through three distinct phases, with corresponding increases in negative and positive reactions. Firstly, the phase of *orientation* where the technical task is the sharing and discovery of information relevant to the problem. Secondly, *evaluation* where the interaction is about the expression of feelings, value judgements and emotional reactions to the information. Thirdly, *control* where the interaction is mainly concerned with suggestions for action, directions, guidance, etc. Negative and positive feelings are present all the time, but the former reach a peak in the third stage followed by a period of positive interchange, presumably to ensure cohesion, face saving and continued attachment to the group. The community worker may have a useful role in facilitating movement of the group through these three phases of decision making.

The Nature and Power of Influence. The second aspect of group decision making is the *nature of power and influence* in the group. We have noted that even leaderless groups devoted to the notion of equal participation will quickly produce a hierarchical structure of influential people, who talk more and take on specialised roles. What then is the basis of power in groups?

French and Raven[25] have examined the different types of relationships between individuals which are the source of particular kinds of power, and have defined five types which seem to them common and important. Their first type is *reward power*, where a group member may be in a position to reward others for certain kinds of conformity: 'If you agree with my view in this instance, I can offer you an important role in executing the decision.' The strength of power increases with the magnitude or salience of the rewards perceived by those others to be available in the situation.

Secondly, they postulated that *coercive power* could be used in a group. Some members will hesitate to disagree with others because they fear punishment by ridicule or being ignored. These types of influence do not lead to any internal change of attitude. Thirdly, there is the complex concept of *legitimate power*, the influence wielded by those who have reached an ascribed or achieved position in the group, backed by the group norm – for example an elected chairman or officer, or a member with considerable status originating in another group or neighbourhood activity. Fourthly, there is the influence of *referent power*, often wielded by an attractive or popular member. There is a desire to be like or closely associated with another, and therefore an inner thrust to adopt their views, attitudes and decisions. Finally, we have the concept of *expert power*, where the influence is mainly felt at a cognitive level as members perceive the power wielder to have more information or experience than they have in certain areas.

The Force of Irrationality. In an attempt to understand why some groups spend a great proportion of time on non-task interactions with evident silent collusion or approval of the members, W. R. Bion[26] has created a profound and fascinating general theory of group behaviour. He speculates that all groups are involved simultaneously in two modes of activity which he describes as the *work group* and the *basic assumption group*. The work group is the aspect of the group that has to do with the real task, and takes cognisance of its purposes, structures itself appropriately, and selects for leadership roles those members with appropriate skills for the matter in hand and who have the ability to organise the members internally in the distribution of labour according to their individual gifts.

The basic assumption activity he describes as being related to our most basic instinctual drives which motivate primitive social behaviour. He named three different phases of basic assumption life: *dependency* (the need for nurture), *fight/flight* (the need for self-preservation) and *pairing* (the need to reproduce). When a group finds the task too difficult, threatening or confusing the members are forced to regress to defensive behaviour in which they engage with surprising energy and purpose. One example of the dependency mode (which frequently marks the beginning stages of a group and which may be exacerbated by the presence of an 'authoritative person' like a councillor or community worker) is a group where the members all act as if they know nothing, are vulnerable, incoherent and inadequate for the purpose. They seek for one strong individual upon whom they can project their fantasies and wish for omnipotence. There is no testing of or disputing the wisdom of the leader's pronouncements; in fact group members appear to feel they need give him little information about their views or suggestions. In other words they act in a totally unscientific way.

Bion's ideas are too complex to deal with in a brief note but merit close study as they relate primarily to behaviour at the group dimension rather than the study of individual interactions, which sometimes means losing sight of the whole.

The Context or Environment of Decision Making. The fourth element to be considered in decision making is the *context or environment* in which it takes place. This refers to internal pressures which create certain emotional moods in the group which differentially affect decision making, communication, productivity and interpersonal relations. The results of Deutsch's work on the difference in productivity between competitive or co-operative groups is interesting in this respect.[27]

(5) *Group Norms and Reactions to Deviance in Groups*
For many people, conformity often has a negative connotation, although many studies of group behaviour have stressed the inevitability and in many cases the usefulness of the development in a group of conformity to its norms. Ongoing groups appear to work at developing a culture, as well as a structure and interpersonal networks. The informal chat phases which mark the beginnings and endings of formal group interaction are, as Brager and Specht[28] have indicated, frequently used by group members to discover attitudes relevant to the work of the group.

Cartwright and Zander[29] have identified four functions of conformity in groups:

to help the group accomplish its goals;
to help the group maintain itself as a group;
to help the members develop validity or 'reality' for their opinions;
to help members define their relations to their social surroundings.

Members identified as leaders in groups carry more weight in norm setting than others. They also appear to be more closely bound by the central norms, partly because their function is to represent the group in outside transactions.[30] The White and Lippitt[31] studies of different leadership style ranging from authoritarian through democratic to *laissez-faire* is a study on the effect on group behaviour of different norms of leader behaviour. With the same groups of children it was found that 'silliness' and inactivity was more prevalent in the *laissez-faire* groups, participation and interdependence in the democratic groups, and low morale, scapegoating and efficiency in the authoritarian groups.

Once adopted by a group, norms have an enduring effect, and this has been demonstrated in a delightful study of children's play groups by Merei.[32] The point for community workers to note in helping groups to recruit and integrate new members is that group traditions and norms are stronger than even the strongest individual, and those aspiring to achieve power must take them into account. They may also be different from the norms of the wider constituency which the group represents and from which it recruits its membership.

Community workers are often concerned to understand the role and dynamics of 'deviance' in community groups. Examples of deviants are the over-talkative member, the domineering chairman, the person who disrupts business by giggling and laughing, the perpetual latecomer, and so forth. There are studies[33] which tell us something about different types of deviants: individuals who deviate, presumably with conscious intent from a position of strength (high status members) and individuals who are 'chosen' by the group to represent an unpopular violation of a norm, who are generally in a position of weakness (low status members). Argyle[34] summarises the reasons why a high status member may deviate. Firstly, the individual may have accepted the influence and adopted the norms of another group in conflict with the goals or values of his group. Secondly, he may have strong individual needs which prevent him accepting some valued norms. Thirdly, he may have arrived at a different set of ideas from the group about how to handle the task. This person may become an innovative deviant and increase his value to the group (if he is allowed to test out his ideas and they work). Or he may have joined the group in order to change its goal or means to a goal. Finally, the deviant may simply wish to challenge the leadership, from motives of rivalry, envy, ambition or dissatisfaction.

It is clear that the presence of a deviant or deviant subgroup is not by any means always dysfunctional. The deviants help the group to identify various boundaries, they prevent rigidity and ossification of ways of working and behaving and may help the group keep in touch with a changing environment which often implies a changed goal.

Low status members who deviate or are 'chosen' (and 'choose') to be scapegoats are not well served by groups and occupy a vulnerable position in groups. Many group theorists suggest that the need to allocate a member to the role of scapegoat is a primary one. The scapegoat is normally a member from whom retaliation is not feared, and there appears to be some weakness of identity present, in that the person appears too readily to accept the projections of others. The function of this phenomenon appears to be to free the other group members from tension and produce a psychic comfort. Low status deviants seem to be selected because of some visible difference (colour, size, disfigurement); because they have little power and an unvalued role in the group; and because they share some common characteristic with a more powerful but feared member. Garland and Kolodny[35] postulate that the scapegoat will commonly show these characteristics: an inability to handle aggression, confused sexual identity, guilt-ridden personality, and attention-seeking behaviour.

In the resolution of conflict in groups it must be noted that violence is more likely to appear in some situations than others. Coser[36] points out that the multiple group memberships experienced by most middle-class individuals offer safety valves for the expression of a variety of different views. Ghetto dwellers, and some other groups such as institutionalised individuals, interact with comparatively few people. Conflict, when one has few or no reference groups as an escape, tends to be intensive. There is also more danger for the deviant in an unorganised group, partly because there is no clear way available for that group to make demands on other groups or institutions and thus release intragroup tension by directing aggression outside. This point leads us to the next section as recent studies indicate that different types of deviancy, problems of integration and conflict resolution arise at different times in a group's history.

(6) Stages of Group Development
The development of a group has been studied both from the perspective of the individual joining and moving through a series of roles until he represents the group and also from a perspective of the total group acquiring different structures, interactional patterns, norms and group consciousness in the drive towards goal achievement.

Mills[37] examines the history of groups from the perspective of different successive orders of group purposes, and the requirements these impose on the role taking of the individuals involved, coupled with the critical issues the group must resolve before moving on to the next and higher stage. Briefly, the stages are as follows:

Stage 1. The purpose of this stage is the immediate gratification of personal needs through interaction with one another, or directly from one another.

Stage 2. The purpose is that of sustaining the group as a source of satisfaction of needs.

Stage 3. The purpose is the pursuit of a collective goal identified by the group.

Stage 4. The fourth stage purpose is self-determination for the group. Members seek to establish relations with a wider environment which will permit them to select their own goals.

Stage 5. The purpose is that of group growth in capabilities, influence and effectiveness in exchange with others.

Examining the stages of group life from the perspective of the totality rather than the individual we find several useful models. Perhaps the best known are Tuckman's[38] stages of forming, storming, norming and performing. Sarri and Galinski[39] have conceptualised a seven stage model which is a fairly typical example. The stages are:

Origin phase. This refers to the composition of the group and motivation for formation which has a significant later effect.

Formative phase. If satisfactory conditions are not established in this phase there will be failure of members to attend. The activities are directed towards seeking common attitudes and objectives. A quasi-structure emerges, often with the most dominant talker seeking and acquiring leadership.

Intermediate stages (1). Group emotional ties are evident; roles are differentiated. A goal has been established and members begin to work towards that. Cliques and subgroups emerge.

Revision. The leadership of the earlier stages is challenged, particularly if the initial leaders have been aggressive and forceful. There may be a change in power builders in the group. Group culture will change if the structure is revised. This is a time of high risk for the group and there is an increase in negative reactions.

Intermediate (2). Equilibrium is restored and often the group is strengthened by the emergence of individuals who have more to contribute to the goals than the initial leaders. Norms are clearer and group cohesion increases. It may be difficult to introduce new members at this stage.

Maturation. Marks a high level of group functioning, with a well developed flexible structure, responsive to environmental demands and opportunities. This is a stage of 'dynamic equilibrium' as the group structure has to adapt to crises emanating from inside or outside the group.

Termination. There appear to be four conditions which result in termination: (1) the goals are attained; (2) essential conditions for endurance are not established (e.g. consensus about goals); (3) the group was planned to endure for a specific time; and (4) maladaptation – the group is unable to respond effectively to external pressures to change.

Finally, community workers will find a useful analysis of different tasks, interactional and technical, appropriate to the different phases of organising in Brager and Specht.[40] The stages are conceptualised as, firstly, that of *socialisation*, when the tasks include the identification and definition of problems and the recruitment and education of potential members;

secondly, the stage of *primary groups*, when the primary tasks are the linking of problems identified to goal development, and fostering social and group cohesion; and thirdly, the stage of *organisation development*, whose purpose is to stabilise the executive function of community members in achieving change. The tasks are those of developing programme objectives and organisation structures, as well as broadening the constituency and developing leadership via building coalitions. These purposes require different skills and personalities and it may well be the most effective course to have changes among the group's membership at different stages.

There are certain problems to be faced by the professional in applying knowledge about phases of group development. For example, what effect do his role-taking and characteristic interventions have on the group? Given that most community workers would attempt to take a boundary role, facilitating the development of natural leaders, the group's progress may be accelerated or diminished appropriately by the actions of this artificial member.

CONCLUSIONS

It is evident from this brief summary that the results of empirical research into small group behaviour present the community worker with a confusing array of data when confronted with his group. One way of ordering the data would be to concentrate on the two aspects of group life frequently mentioned in this paper, the task aspect and the socio-emotional aspect. An important function of a professional working with a group is to monitor the balance and interrelationship between these two aspects. His interventions should then be guided by his assessment. For example, a member who has been related to as a deviant during a meeting may on reflection appear to be the only individual prepared to struggle with a difficult or complex task pertaining to future work, while the group as a whole prefer to bask too long in the pleasant atmosphere of recapitulation of past achievements.

The pressures in a group frequently stem from events or institutions in the environment. In the next section we review some recent thinking on intergroup perceptions and behaviour.

PART TWO: INTERGROUP BEHAVIOUR

In order to survive as an entity a small group must remain in touch with its environment and be responsive to changes in the outside world. The environment of a community group can be exceedingly complex. For example, it must take into account the work processes, values and current events in quite a number of local and even national organisations; social service, health, housing and education departments may simultaneously be targets of a tenant's association seeking to enhance its neighbourhood. Allies in the work for change may well be found in the local religious and voluntary organisations. The tenants' association must of course continue to represent its constituency of a large group of residents, many of whom will be indifferent or apathetic about their plans. The association may well belong to a federation of similar groups and thus be involved in activities with a wider aim than neighbourhood improvement. All these groups must be communicated with, understood, challenged, involved and monitored.

The subject of intergroup behaviour has not as yet attracted a large literature, although of course it is implicit in many sociological, political and historical studies. We shall explore three aspects of intergroup behaviour: the concept of leadership as a boundary function; some problems involved in representing a group to others; intergroup perceptions and conflict.

LEADERSHIP AND THE BOUNDARY

The very many studies on group leadership in recent years suggest that leadership roles arise as a result of individual personality, the social situation, and of the two in interaction. The effective leader of intergroup transactions is the mediator between the inner world of the group and the outer reality of the environment. In relation to its environment the group functions demanded are: the translation of goals into tasks; the identification of necessary resources within and outside the group; the formation of a policy towards the relevant environmental groups; and the monitoring of the steps taken to execute that policy. Quite frequently those functions are divided into parts and assigned to, or taken on by, individual members. However, there may well be a tendency to fragmentation unless the individuals (or subgroups) who oversee the process have the capacity to grasp the relation of the tasks to the ultimate goal.

Leadership roles emerge for individuals who most closely embody the culture and norms of the group and are capable of representing them in the outside world. Another important aspect of leadership is the ability to perceive and understand the culture of other groups, and to modify or hide consequently unhelpful aspects of one's own group culture. This requires intelligence, information and flexibility. Miller and Rice[41] remind us that the task activities and sentience of a group relate to both the inner and outer worlds. The leader's role as a boundary function thus requires that the sentience is understood, accepted and valued, but constantly weighed up as a force which could be advantageous or destructive to the group's endeavours to achieve change.

PROBLEMS OF REPRESENTATION

In order to have intergroup transactions, groups need to have some means of communication as a group and some kind of machinery to enable the choice of the most appropriate representatives. It may well be that the effective manager of intragroup processes is not the best person for negotiation with the outside world. Studies of simulated intergroup transactions (A. K. Rice; G. Higgins and H. Bridger)[42] indicate that representatives can be chosen by most irrational means. The motivation sometimes appears to be to get rid of a troublesome member, or to offer an almost certain opportunity to experience failure and diminishment to a disliked member. If a group is in disagreement or confusion about the proposed negotiations those feelings can be manifested in the choice of a pair of delegates who are in disagreement about the task or a person who will effectively communicate the group's confusion about the issues and little else.

Groups can be seduced into choosing representatives by virtue of an individual's position (e.g. chairman), because a tradition has evolved to avoid conflict by having individuals take turns, or simply because an individual was successful on a previous occasion, which in fact demanded very different skills and expertise.

Groups tend to place too little value on the authority with which they back a representative's mandate. Time consuming though the process may be, successful action demands that representatives know the precise limit of their powers in negotiations, particularly as these often involve committing their group to further actions. The model developed by the Tavistock Group[43] consists of three differentiated functions of representation; its simplicity and clarity can be useful.

Observer
The person carrying out this function has sanction only to obtain information from other groups, not to express views or give information about his group's affairs.

Delegate
The representative is empowered to deliver a message, express a (carefully worked out) point of view, or take a specified action on behalf of his group; he has no sanction to vary any of these communications from those agreed by his group, and must refer back to group before making any changes on its behalf.

Plenipotentiary
The representative is empowered to do the best he can in the light of the known views or policies of his group. His terms of reference are flexible; of course he is sometimes given limits beyond which he may not go.

Confusion about the type of brief they carry among members or negotiating groups has had very severe consequences. The Irish Civil War in 1921 arose partly from allegations that Michael Collins and his team in negotiating the treaty with the British Government had acted as plenipotentiaries when the authority given them did not extend beyond that of delegates.

Groups may tend to invest too much energy and interest in their current intergroup transactions, so that business virtually ceases until the results of one particular negotiation are known. If these results are negative the group has no contingency plans or alternative strategies to employ and may waste energy in frustrated and impotent anger. On the other hand, if the group is highly creative in devising a variety of tasks and approaches for its members, it may tend to undervalue the results of protracted negotiation when finally informed of what should be an important gain. The representatives among the group members must complement as allies the managers of the intragroup process, if their work is to be validated and used.

INTERGROUP PERCEPTIONS

No communication takes place between individuals or groups outside a relational context, formed by past experience or future hope or designs. These relational elements between groups appear to be based on fantasy quite as frequently as relations between individuals. Sherif[44] in studies of intergroup behaviour confirms the observations of psychologists and others that individuals tend to idealise important groups they belong to and deny their less attractive features. They tend to attribute less attractive features to other groups and deny their positive ones.

Sherif discusses two traditional practices used in handling intergroup hostility. He found them common, and believed they tended to magnify rather than deal with the problems. Firstly the practice of assigning blame for the hostility. Group members often act in such a way as to make their assumptions about 'enemy' groups into self-fulfilling prophecies. Blame casting and self-justification lead to stereotyped perceptions, and the actions of the hated or feared group may conform to a persistent labelling of them as a hostile one. The relations between some groups of immigrant teenagers and the police are a good example.

The second practice is that of *deterrence* behaviour, used both in international relations and by the teenage groups studied by Sherif: 'Deterrence concepts all assume that one is facing an enemy whose intent is hostile. It is further assumed that the outbreak of violence can be avoided if one or the other can amass superior capabilities to threaten the opponent . . .' Analogous to the banking of nuclear weapons by nations, or green apples by Sherif's teenagers, may be the work of finding allies in activities for

D

and against social change, so that the energy on both sides goes to building fairly useless power blocks.

There are vertical intergroup relations as well as horizontal ones, while there may be quite real differences of opinion between one organisational department and another about the best ways to define and achieve goals. It is a common phenomenon in small group behaviour that anxiety, tension, and conflict are dealt with by projecting blame on an outside group. Frequently this is functional for the cohesion or sentience of the group but disastrous for the tasks in which the various groups should co-operate.

PART THREE: BEHAVIOUR IN LARGE GROUPS

Community workers spend a good deal of their time working with individuals and small groups: committees, tenants' associations, etc. It is likely, however, that they also will find themselves attempting to work (for instance, at a public meeting) with a collectivity where face-to-face interaction is not possible for all the members, and the dynamics of those groups (anything from twenty-five upwards) appear to possess some different properties from those we have discussed. The resulting observations and theorising may provide some guidelines for the community worker attempting to take a member or leader role in a large meeting.

It must be remembered that it is almost impossible to make a scientific study of large group behaviour. Some attempts made to reproduce in a laboratory setting the panic reactions of crowds ended in scientific disaster (detailed in most basic social psychology texts). However there is enough commonality in the observations or speculations of those who have consistently studied or worked with large, unstructured groups to give reasonable validity to their conclusions.

Current writers still draw on the work of Le Bon[45] and Freud[46], however critical they may feel about the ultimate and pessimistic conclusions of these writers. Le Bon was interested in the process of revolution in France and the mobs who appeared to bring about changes. In analysing the behaviour of individuals in crowds he noted (as have practically all other writers on the subject) the increase of emotion, loss of responsibility, release of inhibition and diminishment of the effect of some usual forms of social behaviour.

Collective behaviour as we discuss it must have a goal, or point of focus. Individuals going about their business in the street are presumably not a crowd in this sense. Le Bon defined the actors in collective behaviour as a large number of people with a common objective (which may arise spontaneously), a common object of interest and a feeling for the presence of others like themselves, and a sharing of the experience. What is less clear from the literature is whether these phenomena appear in already structured large groups – an organisation, a congregation in church, the audience at a theatre. Collective behaviour is not institutionalised; it is not governed by established norms. (Sometimes of course in unusually long-lasting episodes of collective behaviour norms do emerge – agreement about objectives and ways of working. An example is the well organised 'rioting' children who attack the British army in the streets of Belfast and Londonderry in the 1970s.) Rather, collective behaviour demands a reasonable consensus and – according to Brown[47] – a belief system: belief in extraordinary forces at work in the world, belief in great dangers, in conspiracies or in golden wish-fulfilling prophecies.

Smelser[48] has systematised the conditions which in his view appear to lead to collective behaviour. His analysis includes both sociological and psychological determinants and emphasise the power of rumour, as opposed to information, in motivating action:

1 Structural conduciveness: certain societal conditions must exist, e.g. institutionalised minority/majority groups such as blacks and whites in America, Catholics and Protestants in Northern Ireland.
2 Structural strain: the existence of dissonance in societal values. In a democracy the minority may not have their needs listened to but must loyally support the majority.
3 Growth and spread of a generalised belief: suspicion, doubt and rumour create widespread fantasies, e.g. all the Catholics in Northern Ireland are conspiring to bring about domination from the South.
4 A precipitating factor: a report (often an exaggerated rumour) of an event which appears to confirm the widespread belief.
5 Mobilisation of participants for action: leaders must emerge around whom groups begin to cluster and whom they will follow. The quality of this leadership is crucial. Some leaders of riots or lynch mobs were later found to be dangerously undersocialised characters. Most observers will agree that the level of thinking in a crowd is usually at an intellectually low level. The leader who wins support will do so by appealing to the emotion of the moment by using deceptively simple analogies and rhetoric. He wins followers who cry for action rather than thought.
6 Inadequate presence or absence of social control forces; ineffective policing or sanctions available.

In a large group individuals have often taken action, or have refrained from action, in ways that cause them later to feel profound guilt. At a surface level the individual is affected by the inevitable defects in communication. Free interchange is absent and the majority are bound to be passive. Half heard, half understood statements go unchallenged; many individuals do not understand what is happening and appear to be much more open than usual to suggestion and influence, carried away perhaps by fantasies about the omnipotence of large numbers of people acting together and a credulous belief in the rightness of the actions.

A more profound level of psychological analysis has been made by group therapists and trainers who have studied large groups of patients or trainees set up for specific purposes but lacking in structures beyond having the services of two or more consultants in group behaviour. Turquet[49] discusses the painful dilemma for the individual in large groups. He suffers a crisis of identity, and has a choice between either withdrawal and self-effacement with the danger of feeling submerged and taken over or expressing his views and feelings, exposing himself to the attack, judgement or misperception of a large number. The stimuli of communication are generally confusing and overwhelming. Before one can take in, assess and respond to one idea or proposal several more have superseded it. Discussion in a large group rarely follows any logical progression. The anxiety created by the situation teaches individuals to come with prepared statements and they tend to use other members as a peg to get in, rather than to listen and respond. Because our identity and self-image appear to need continual reassurance from others the individual searches in vain for a stable small group with which he can interact. This may be the people sitting near by, members of the same sex, colour or ethnic group, neighbours, etc. Experience shows that coalitions of this nature can rarely achieve stability.

Pines[50] suggests some techniques used in psychotherapy in large groups which enabled the group to work in an orderly and rational manner.

One example is the creation of a number of 'representatives' of smaller collections of the individuals present who hold preliminary meetings with their 'constituents' and later give a report of their views and perceptions of events to the meeting, mentioning most individuals by name. This tends to give a form of structure, diminish anonymity and create conditions in which more individuals will feel secure in speaking. Another technique used in educational groups is to deal with the pacing and comprehension of important information by the formation of 'buzz groups', small neighbouring groups of three to six members who remain in the room but take time out to discuss and reach conclusions on the matters to be dealt with. Their conclusions may be shared, a process which slows down the pace and allows for the perception of complexities and different views and approaches. Both these models allow some scope for participation, individual creativity and thought, those basic ingredients of satisfaction for individuals which otherwise is lacking in the large group.

CONCLUSION

Clearly there is a wealth of knowledge about groups, which can be acquired by diligent study. For the student (and trainer) a more difficult task is the integration of this knowledge with his own experience of the 'familiar chaos' (as Homans nicely puts it) of group behaviour. A welcome development is the workshop or 'laboratory' method of training, in which experiences can be structured to an extent that the learner can build up his own concepts, and develop his own framework for knowing and acting. In the last analysis the community worker must decide for himself which of the theories he adopts stand up to the test of his reality.

REFERENCES

1 D. Cartwright and A. Zander, *Group Dynamics: Research & Theory* (London, Tavistock Publications, 1968), p. 46.
2 E. Bott, *Family and Social Network*, 2nd edn (London, Tavistock Publications, 1971), chapters 6 and 7.
3 N. W. Bell and E. F. Vogel, *A Modern Introduction to the Family* (New York, Free Press, 1968), Part 2.
4 G. Coyle, 'Concepts Relevant to helping the family as a Group', in E. Younghusband (ed.), *Social Work with Families* (London, George Allen & Unwin, 1965).
5 M. Phillips, *Small Social Groups in England* (London, Methuen, 1965).
6 R. F. Bales, 'Task Roles and Social Roles in Problem-solving Groups' in E. Maccoby, T. M. Newcomb and E. L. Hartley (eds), *Readings in Social Psychology*, 3rd edn. (London, Methuen, 1961).
7 D. Cartwright and A. Zander, op. cit., p. 56.
8 A. H. Maslow, *Motivation and Personality* (New York, Harper & Row, 1954), pp. 80–108.
9 D. Cartwright and A. Zander, op. cit., pp. 401–7.
10 B. H. Raven and J. Rietsema, 'The Effects of Varied Clarity of Group Goal and Group Path, on the Individual and his relation to the Group' in D. Cartwright and A. Zander, *Group Dynamics*, 2nd edn (London, Tavistock, 1966).
11 W. F. Whyte, *Street Corner Society* (Chicago, University of Chicago Press, 1943).
12 G. C. Homans, *The Human Group* (London, Routledge & Kegan Paul, 1951).
13 J. L. Moreno, *Who Shall Survive* (Washington D.C., Nervous & Mental Disease Publishing Company, 1934).
14 H. H. Jennings, *Leadership and Isolation* (New York, McKay, 1943).
15 R. F. Bales, 'Task Roles & Social Roles in Problem-solving Groups', op. cit.
16 R. F. Bales and P. E. Slater, 'Role differentiation in small decision-making Groups' in T. Parsons and R. F. Bales (eds), *The Family Socialization & Interaction Process* (New York, Free Press, 1955).
17 D. N. Thomas, *Organising for Social Change: A Study in the Theory and Practice of Community Work* (London, George Allen & Unwin, 1976), chapter 6.

18 M. Argyle, *Bodily Communication* (London, Methuen, 1975), Part 2.
19 S. Alinsky, *Rules for Radicals* (New York, Random House, 1971), pp. 70–1.
20 B. Bernstein, 'Some Sociological Determinants of Perception' in *British Journal of Sociology*, volume 9 (1958).
21 D. N. Thomas, op. cit., p. 120.
22 R. F. Bales, 'Task Roles and Social Roles in Problem-solving Groups', op. cit.
23 A. Bavelas, 'Communication Patterns in Task-oriented Groups' in Cartwright and Zander, op. cit., pp. 503–11.
24 R. F. Bales and F. L. Strodtbeck, 'Phases in Group Problem-solving' D. Cartwright and A. Zander, op. cit., pp. 389–98.
25 J. R. P. French and B. Raven, 'The Bases of Social Power', in Cartwright and Zander, op. cit., pp. 259–69.
26 W. R. Bion, *Experiences in Groups* (London, Tavistock, 1961).
27 M. Deutsch, 'The Effects of Cooperation and Competition upon Group Process' in Cartwright and Zander, op. cit., pp. 461–82.
28 G. Brager and H. Specht, *Community Organizing* (New York, Columbia University Press, 1973), pp. 118–22.
29 D. Cartwright and A. Zander, op. cit., p. 142.
30 G. C. Homans, op. cit., chapters 7 and 8.
31 R. White and R. Lippett, 'Leader Behaviour and Member Reaction in Three Social Climates' in Cartwright and Zander, op. cit., pp. 318–35.
32 F. Merei, 'Group Leadership and Institutionalization', in E. E. Maccoby, T. M. Newcomb and E. L. Hartley (eds), *Readings in Social Psychology* (London, Methuen, 1961), pp. 522–31.
33 See for example G. C. Homans, op. cit., chapters 7 and 8; S. Schachter, 'Deviation, Rejection and Communication' in Cartwright and Zander, op. cit., pp. 165–81.
34 M. Argyle, *Social Interaction* (London, Methuen, 1969), p. 226.
35 J. A. Garland and R. L. Kolodny, 'The Characteristics and Resolution of Scapegoating', in S. Bernstein (ed.), *Further Explorations in Group Work* (London, Bookstall, 1972).
36 L. S. Coser, *Continuities in the study of Social Conflict* (London, Collier-Macmillan, 1967).
37 T. M. Mills, *The Sociology of Small Groups* (New Jersey, Prentice Hall, 1967), chapter 7.
38 B. Tuckman, 'Development Sequence in Small Groups', in *Psychological Bulletin* 1963, pp. 384–99.
39 R. C. Sarri and M. J. Galinski, 'A Conceptual Framework for Group Development', in P. Glasser, R. C. Sarri and R. Vinter (eds), *Individual Change through Small Groups* (New York, Free Press, 1974).
40 G. Brager and H. Specht, op. cit., chapters 4, 5, 6 and 7.
41 E. Miller and A. K. Rice, *Systems of Organization* (London, Tavistock, 1967), chapter 1.
42 A. K. Rice, *Learning for Leadership* (London, Tavistock, 1965), chapter 7, and G. Higgin and H. Bridger, 'Psychodynamics of an Inter-group Exercise' in *Journal of Human Relations*, 1964, vol. 17, No. 4, pp. 391–444.
43 A. K. Rice, op. cit., pp. 92–7.

44 M. Sherif, *Group Conflict and Co-operation* (London, Routledge & Kegan Paul, 1967), chapter 7.
45 G. Lebon, *The Crowd* (London, Ernest Benn, 1896).
46 S. Freud, *Group Psychology and the Analysis of the Ego* (London, Hogarth, 1922).
47 R. Brown, *Social Psychology* (New York, Free Press, 1965), chapter 14.
48 N. J. Smelser, *Theory of Collective Behaviour* (New York, Free Press, 1963.)
49 P. Turquet, 'Threats to Identity in the Large Group' in L. Kreeger (ed.), *The Large Group* (London, Constable, 1975), pp. 87–144.
50 M. Pines, 'Overview' in L. Kreeger, op. cit.

Chapter 7

PUTTING THINGS INTO PERSPECTIVE: RESEARCH METHODS AND COMMUNITY WORK

John Lambert

A great deal of social research seems to consist in extraordinary elaborations of the obvious; and much policy research seems to operate with an assumption that the world will change if a well researched inquiry proves the need for change. Community workers are well placed to know that the relationship between knowledge, facts and action is problematical; and they will rightly be sceptical about the contribution of research because of the way research – so expensive of time and funds – can be used as an alternative to action, as a form of delay and diversion. However, criticisms of research and researchers should not be allowed to detract from the advantages a research approach and some research methods can have for community workers in setting about their tasks.

The qualities which the dictionary[1] definition of research points to are those of *care* in a search of inquiry, of *science* guiding the endeavour of discovery, and of *criticism* informing any investigation. Those qualities sound unambiguously like components community work should share with research. In a good piece of research the methods whereby the researcher proceeded are transparent. In effect the researcher is saying that 'anyone who followed these methods would reach the same conclusions'. It is by reference to his methods not to his ideology, beliefs or other factors that the researcher claims legitimacy: replicability ensures objectivity. This also sounds like a good basis for community work.

RESEARCH AND ACTION

However, these very qualities contribute to the tension which undoubtedly exists between research and action. *Care* and insistence on method can mean that the researcher needs time and must not be hurried, whereas the community worker may need to know fast; next week's meeting is a crucial deadline at which something must be said and at which decisions will be taken willy-nilly. About the *scientific* nature of social inquiry there is of course a considerable debate to which we will return later, but people are not objects and a neighbourhood is not a laboratory; facts don't necessarily speak for themselves and the claim that methods can be divorced from the values and ideology of the person employing them is to be doubted. *Critical investigation* can elaborate on the nature of questions and answers and aid rather than remove difficult decisions about what is to be done.

So research methods and skills can suggest ways of proceeding for a community worker; they can contribute to debate and discussion over matters of strategy and value. A research approach can be a starting-point for a community worker to enter into a dialogue which may result in action. I would suggest that community workers by nature of their involvement are well placed to 'do research' on community problems and issues and so improve their own and residents' understanding of the situation. What underlies much of the tension between research and action is that traditionally and conveniently research is sponsored by the powerful and its findings, if used at all, are in a form that is intelligible to the sponsors. Research findings are not neutral since intelligence and understanding are a part of control and power. But by the same token the procedures of research can be utilised by a wider public. The use a community worker makes of findings is a question that will be answered by reference to the worker's aims, interests and values; an answer does not rest within the research.

RESEARCH APPROACHES IN CURRENT COMMUNITY WORK

Many projects in community work incorporate some elements of a research approach. Notwithstanding the lottery character of much community work funding (especially Urban Aid) there would seem to be a fairly clear consensus about what makes a good grant application: a demonstration of need, a realistic appraisal of solutions, a set of operations which link solutions and need, and a demonstration of competence. An appeal to some research findings relevant to the topic or locality is a sensible component of any grant application.

Less common, but perhaps likely to be stressed in future, are attempts to analyse and evaluate projects (to demonstrate perhaps that sponsors are getting 'value for money'). The most recent Gulbenkian Report[2] offers a first outline or framework for such an analysis. The suggested approach adapts the experimental model of social research: statement of objectives, formulation of hypotheses, description of intended operations, recording of process, observation of outcome, presentation of findings. Such an approach requires of a worker a well developed research perspective and at the moment is more likely to be a source of anxiety to staff and students on training courses than to be put into action in the hurly-burly of neighbourhood community work.

There are ways in which a research approach can be simply a way of starting for a community worker new to an area; a reason for interviewing and so meeting local people or officials can be gained from initiating an unpretentious study or research project. However, the community worker initiating any study needs to take care that no one else has been around recently asking similar questions for one of the many official and unofficial bodies which engage in surveys and studies. And if the aim is not so much findings as contacts and discussions to suggest other lines of action, then the caution is doubly necessary. A community worker needs to be able to assess the policy aims, claims and outcomes affecting a neighbourhood. Such policies may utilise research reports, surveys and findings. So there is value in the community worker as *research consumer* being knowledgeable about the rules of the research game or the tricks of the research trade if he is to do other than accept the findings. As a *research practitioner* a worker will need to know about, and be able to exploit, existing sources of data about his area or topic of interest, and he will need to know how best to manufacture the knowledge his group needs to sustain its argument or position.

Ashcroft and Jackson[3] report on a piece of community work which entailed their preparing, for discussion at a public meeting and in small groups, a document 'aiming to produce a full and reasoned statement about [the] purpose, nature and context' of the 1972 Housing Finance Act. Their article does not elaborate on the procedures involved in constructing such a paper – we are told that it ran to five sides of duplicated paper and took one hour to present. Very few community workers (or any other sort of worker) in my experience would know where to begin such a task: clearly its construction required the scrutiny of documents, the careful search for relevant background content, a presentation of facts which sustained an argument and the critical application of findings to a specific locale. Accompanying it was a concern for clear logical presentation in a language and form that achieved communication to a specific audience. All the components, indeed, of a research approach.

In 'The Sparkbrook West Story'[4] it is reported that the local council responded to some demands from a residents' association by asking for evidence that there was genuine interest in improvement as against redevelopment in parts of an area where planning proposals were in preparation. Within a month the association was able to organise an effective total survey of two specified areas and report findings to the city's planning department. The community worker with this association had some experience of research methods and was able to point out some of the difficulties; more important was some previous experience of those residents active in the association who had done an earlier survey and discovered the difficulties in making contact and collecting information from people in a neighbourhood. When it mattered, however, they were prepared for the task and in subsequent negotiations both the speed and the effectiveness of their surveys gave them evidence which was both in a form the planners were used to having and had a legitimacy in their terms for the case the residents wished to argue.

Community work and community workers are sometimes accused of dealing with trivial local issues or of lacking an awareness of the broader context for such local issues. One valuable result of some of the Community Development Projects is the utilisation of research – funded on a scale unlikely to be possible for most community work projects – for community work. A report like 'Workers on the Scrap Heap'[5] is particularly interesting. It explores carefully the nature of the industrial and employment blight which lay behind the more familiar physical and community blight which beset the project area. It needed a person with time to piece together somewhat inaccessible but not confidential information and with care, science and criticism present some findings. No obvious solutions, however, emerge to spark off a new style community work campaign in the area. But to expect such from a research document would be mistaken. Research for community work is part of an input to debate and discussion on strategy and aims; it provides no substitutes for that debate or discussion.

These, then, are some ways in which research methods and their application can become a valuable and perhaps essential part of a community work enterprise. I have tried to suggest that research is not unambiguously a community worker's best friend and if a worker is not to be blinded by the science of professional research he will need to get wise to the scope and style and limitations of research practice. In the next part of this chapter, I want to look at certain features of different methods and point to ways in which they may be used by community workers.

METHOD IN RESEARCH

There is a need to distinguish how research is presented from how it is practised. Textbooks on research methods[6] frequently introduce a paradigm of the scientific method for social inquiry: theory–hypothesis–test– confirm or falsify hypothesis–accept or modify theory. This suggests a neatness which is invariably impossible in research practice; it implies a logic which is invaluable when reporting on research undertaken.

In real life a topic or problem crops up and debate leads to inquiry. The researcher looks around for material relevant to the topic and is likely to be on the watch for contrary signs or for a reason to modify his original conceptualisation. He will record what he did so as to be able to retrace his steps and identify his choices along the way. In presenting his findings he may however choose not to recount all the procedures, blind alleys and about turns but to select those elements which at the end of the day proved most reliable. Replicability depends more on a series of logical sequences than on any exact repeat of all procedures.

The paradigm of the hypothetico-deductive system for social research is not intended to lay down for research rigidities in procedure which may be appropriate, say, for scientific experiments of a routine sort in the controlled environment of a laboratory. Research is a matter of searching around for evidence and materials, of being open to new ideas, of redefining problems, of continuous questioning. Where discipline and rigidity enter is in the recording process, selecting and presenting themes and in the drawing of conclusions. The researcher needs to be able to demonstrate how he reached his conclusions and implicitly suggests that anyone following the methods he presents would reach the same conclusions. He will appeal to rules and conventions, cautions and safeguards which experience and practice have devised for a number of different styles of research methodology. At different stages one research project may utilise various styles and various data. In the following sections some of these are reviewed for community workers.

Participant Observation
This research style is probably the most natural for the community worker but properly done it only *seems* like hanging about and doing nothing. It is easy for it to remain on a glib and superficial level. To go beyond, it needs to be rigorously organised and disciplined and, when subject to the critical demands of a research approach, it can yield a breadth and depth of knowledge of great usefulness.

Researchers and community workers have rather different opportunities for observations, visits, following up contacts, informal interviewing, and the like. The researcher with no long-term interest in involvement is freer to experiment with all sorts of ploys and disguises to get into interesting situations. The community worker with a clearer and continuing identity may be more limited in scope. An awareness of how some scenes are closed off from view and how the observer is influencing a situation is crucial for research based on seemingly casual observations and visits.

Such observations and visits can be valuable sources of data, but only to the extent that the researcher can treat critically what he finds out. What were his prior definitions of the situation? In what way were they confirmed or countered by his informants? What did he know about his informants and what were his assumptions about them? If they were professionals and outsiders, in what way was their involvement influencing their definitions of the situation? Such questions are the kind with which a researcher will confront his observational findings in order to piece together the nature of *his* developing perspective on the thing being observed.

A necessary aspect of observation is the way records of observations are maintained. No researcher or community worker can go about with notebook or tape recorder and record all that happens; not, that is, unless he wishes to attract attention to himself and obtain information of a different sort. Memories are notoriously selective in their capacity to hold significant occasions in detail. Researchers probably adopt numerous different procedures for recording observations. Most would probably remember at the outset how they underestimated the time it takes to report or record 'what happened' yet, without adequate recording, making sense of the data – or, more correctly, turning observations into data to make sense of – will be extremely partial and subjective.[7]

Using Existing Sources of Data
There is an extraordinary variety of official and semi-official data sources on all sorts of topics.[8] A careful reading of newspapers will show these sources being used for news stories and it is indeed the case that an enormous amount of background and context material exists if only researchers and community workers know where to locate it. Great care has to be taken in utilising such material for the mode of collection can lead to a wholly spurious exactitude. Frequently the data is only recorded for, it seems, the sake of recording and may mix up careful assessments with hurried 'guesstimates', depending on who was responsible, and where, for the data collection. Researchers need to know how the data sources were made before they can be used reliably for research purposes and it is a caution community workers should observe as well.

These data sources are of limited use for community workers since they rarely relate to small areas such as a neighbourhood. Sometimes local councils compile special abstracts of local statistics which will provide information for each local ward, but these may still be large and diverse areas. The Census is published for a whole variety of area sizes from ward to region but is built up from data sources for extremely small areas – enumeration districts of just a few streets. This small area data is provided to local councils and to some university departments, and researchers and community workers can usefully get to know where such data is kept and whether special analysis or studies can be made. Such analysis can be time-consuming and low on productivity and best utilised only after obtaining good advice.

Such advice probably holds for a lot of official sources which can be opaque and misleading except to real *aficionados* of the data source game. Getting to know such experts may bring a quicker pay-off for a community worker than actually tackling the tomes of figures directly.

Other existing sources of data on a particular locality rest in libraries in all manner of documents, books and reports. Again these are records created for purposes other than research and their original purpose should be borne in mind. 'Content analysis' is the term for a variety of techniques social research has devised to achieve rigorous exploitation of such sources. At its simplest this consists in noting and quantifying themes which recur in the accounts, say, of local newspaper editorials or in letters to the editor. More elaborate systems can be evolved for constructing categories for classifying different treatment of themes. Such methods would ordinarily only be utilised if the documentary records were ample and complete and for a particularly focused study. For a community worker seeking an orientation or a perspective to local problems and issues such methods allow a way of treating systematically and critically a variety of sources.

Using Surveys

The survey is probably the most common, most abused, but – properly used – the most valuable method of social research for community workers. Textbooks tend to reflect the domination of the survey-research field by market research: a somewhat pretentious pseudotechnology using vast resources of personnel and hardware has grown up to organise mass surveys. Fortunately, community workers are unlikely ever to have the resources for such efforts and can ignore the minutiae and sophisticated guidelines of the textbooks. A simpler model of the survey can prevail and the notion of the 'community self-survey', once popular, can perhaps be revived.

Essentially a survey is the systematic asking of questions or noticing behavioural responses of a definite population or audience. It is a system for gathering data economically from a large population. Providing a random (i.e. scientifically devised and calculated) sample of the population is interviewed, the characteristics of the whole population can be inferred within limits of confidence reasonable enough for most practical purposes. If it is known that the population is fairly uniform on some variables relevant to the studied variable then it is safe to take quite a small sample – 1 in 20 perhaps. If little is known about the population or if it is known to be heterogeneous then a larger sample will be advisable, perhaps 1 in 5 or 1 in 10. In practice is it often wiser to calculate the number of interviews possible from the number of interviewers available and select *systematically* (i.e. randomly) families or homes for that number of interviews.

Since the survey depends on a number of interviewers, care must be taken to see that they are drilled to do the same thing. The textbooks are full of hints about correct uniform wording and order of questions. The survey method presumes that interviewer and respondent can tacitly agree on some common ground on which unambiguous and honest discourse can occur. Different people have different views on the extent of that common ground: barriers of class and language can play havoc with surveyors' hopes and assumptions. The textbooks are full of warnings about the ease with which surveyors can impose language values and interests and unconsciously force respondents into answering not on some common ground but on the ground of the surveyor. If this sounds abstract then would-be surveyors should test for themselves just how easy it is to vary responses by using different words, by shifts in manner and by contrasting conversational interviews with no fixed order of questions with the familiar closed question schedule.

Consistent with the mass character of the survey, a particular type of response is sought: one that can be coded. Again textbooks and handbooks are full of useful tips about the construction and formulation of answer types and categories. It is not useful to have answers which are long sentences unless there is time enough to submit them to a content analysis. It is also an area where different interviewers can record answers so differently that the aims of a systematic survey can be defeated.

Some other essentials for good community surveys are as follows:

the necessity always to do a trial run or pilot to check on the language, length and intelligibility of the survey;
to remember that non-respondents and refusers are likely to be different from respondents and must be remembered in any analysis;
the temptation to add odd questions 'just for interest' should be resisted. The best surveys are short and focused, and inexperienced surveyors grossly underestimate the time it takes to make sense of coded or verbatim answers.

The question of who shall do the interviewing is an important one for community workers. Few community worker projects are likely to be in a position to employ professionals and most will use students or local activists. It can be argued that a cool, detached, neutral doorstep rapport may be easier to organise with students than with neighbours. Residents are more likely to suggest a sensible and common-language formulation of questions and overcome some of the problems of non-response. However, it should not be assumed that neighbours will find it natural and easy to call on one another and ask questions unless all are utterly convinced of the need for a proper survey. I wonder how many eager surveying community workers have wondered what to do with an interviewer who reports satisfactory completion of all schedules but adds: 'Jim S. wasn't in but I filled it in all the same because I know just how he feels', and a little later says: 'Of course I didn't bother calling at 37 and 55 – they're Pakistanis.'

Interviewing
The survey adapts the interview for a situation in which a number of interviewers question a large audience. Social research has formulated considerable techniques to organise and structure the deceptively straightforward art of interviewing. Community workers can be well advised to study one of the many handbooks with suggestions for organising inter-

views. The quest is for unobtrusive organisation whereby the interviewee covers the topics the interviewer reckons important without the interviewee being aware of it, and whereby the interviewee is prevented from expatiating on his chosen topics which *may* be irrelevant for the interviewer (they may, however, be precisely what the interview is all about). Interviewing can adopt many styles which depend on who is being interviewed and how the interviewer is seen: sometimes a detailed schedule will be advisable; at others a discussion of a prepared checklist of topics; at others the form will be of an open-ended discussion when a checklist of topics is in the interviewer's head. Recording responses is a great problem. Few people like to have someone taking down what they say in a notebook; sometimes if a second person can accompany the interviewer unobtrusive notetaking can be arranged. Otherwise memory has to be trusted and the period between the interview and writing it up should be as short as possible (consecutive interviews are dangerous because of the ease with which the memory can muddle up who said what). The emergence of small cassette recorders with built-in sensitive microphones makes unobtrusive recording of interviews much more possible. Such recorders can be invaluable in attaining a very rapid review of an unrecorded interview more quickly and conveniently than writing it down on paper.

In obtaining interviews researchers can usually appeal to the ideal of research and flatter respondents into contributing to pushing forward the frontiers of knowledge. The community worker may have to resort at times to ploys both more honest and more devious if there is purpose enough in having someone spill some relevant beans. It is easy to assume that interviewing is simple and straightforward, but in exploiting the full potential of the interview community workers should certainly study the techniques developed in social research.

Investigations

Survey methods can be the manipulation of a powerless and unsuspecting audience for ends that are opaque and with results that rarely get back to the providers of the data. The purpose of much of the artistry and technique developed for interviewing is to ease the collection of data from persons assumed to be both powerful and suspecting. There is an emerging field of social research which is seeking to investigate people in other ways: the exploration of institutions, agencies, companies and individuals in a way which may be indirect but which seeks to exploit and organise what is publicly knowable about such bodies.

Such investigations are indeed part of community action and a radical sociology which rejects the ideological loadings of conventional research methods. Such investigatory techniques combine the care and the rigour and the concern for documentation of conventional research with the concerns of local politics and trade unions in a style that owes much to investigatory journalism. Conventional research trains students for elaborate negotiations with working-class respondents (or more likely their wives) on doorsteps but says very little in the way of finding out about the nature of the controlling institutions. However, through such agencies as *Counter Information Services* and *Community Action*, a new style of social research is emerging. *Community Action's* 'Investigators Handbook' is a first attempt at a guide to methods and sources of information.[9]

For community workers seeking to gain an understanding of a locality and its issues and where it stands, such inquiries are probably a first starting-point. A worker will be led into sources of data and avenues which conventional social research scarcely touches. The concern for care, science and criticism which guide research are no less applicable here.

The Communication of Findings

In all these methods and styles the need to record carefully and systematically has been stressed. Writing things down clearly is a part of social research so obvious that it can easily be overlooked and taken for granted; it becomes crucial for the clear and unambiguous presentation of findings. The art of clear expression is no more common among social researchers than among any other group of professionals and it consists of skills difficult, if not impossible, to learn or teach. The logic of the scientific method is supposedly a simple and ideal form but, as with the practices and procedures of inquiry, so the reality of research findings and presentation is often tortuous and obfuscating. For the community worker there are added problems in that his audience or public may not have the time and sophistication to grapple with sets of figures and complex argument. It should be a skill of research to know ways of presenting figures in diagrammatic and pictorial form, of explaining – not merely presenting – statistics and of reducing the complexities of arguments to essentials. In practice such skills are rare. Other areas of community work training – the exploitation of video and other media techniques – have ways of making findings of research activity intelligible and meaningful for a neighbourhood group or organisation.

EMPIRICISM, IDEOLOGY AND THE NATURE OF SOCIAL INNOVATION

Of the qualities of care, criticism and science, the first two have been stressed in relation to all of the styles and methods of research discussed in the previous section. The claim for the nature of social inquiry as scientific is problematical, however, and in this final section the nature of the problem must be tackled, albeit superficially.

The task of proper method is to obtain good data. The data sources of social research are ultimately people. Data derives from recorded impressions of the actual experiences of real people in contact with the 'real world out there'. The aim of research strategy is to catch and record events as facts from which by induction theoretical knowledge is acquired. Empiricism is the term for this procedure whereby observation and experiment precede theory in the acquiring of knowledge. The care and concern in social research for the declaration of value positions and assumptions prompting inquiry, procedures like sampling and content analysis which systematically eradicate biases, and the critical distinction between statements of tendency, probability and of laws are all procedures to control the influence of the researcher on his findings. Those findings are ultimately derived from reported experiences treated, for the purposes of research, as facts.

There is a critique of this empiricism in application to social study which considers that the objectification or facticity of natural science dehumanises the context of social inquiry. The real world is not made up of events except as occurring within a framework of values and ideas; 'facts' are an expression of those ideas and no amount of scientific procedure can achieve the separation of those facts from the values which inhere there. Empiricism and science in relation to social studies treat the appearance and forms and definitions of social reality as given and largely unproblematical. Indeed this borrowing from natural science serves to ignore, conceal or mystify the social nature of the arrangements which lie behind the 'facts'. In study and research on social problems the influence of this scientistic positivism is most marked. Research gathers facts about various categories of need, about the life styles and attitudes of the poor and needy, about criminals and delinquents, crime and delinquency. Attention falls on these subjects as objects and the forms of behaviour tend to be treated as independent from each other and from other 'non-problem' forms. The appearance is accepted for what it is.

There is another approach which treats the events, the data of empirical inquiry, as providing clues about a more significant reality behind 'what seems'. Instead of collecting facts in a refined and value-free way (but with careful and critical attention to method), the task of social research is to analyse the appearances of everyday life, its organisational forms and the meanings which people ascribe to their practice and experience in relation to the dominant but hidden structural relations which control and shape the visible forms of social living. This approach insists on the importance of a *class* analysis to relate the everyday forms, the appearances, to the dominant ideas about social order. Social reality is studied to reveal the workings-out of dominant or ruling-class ideas. This approach may sound dauntingly political to some community workers or merely a debunking exercise with no relationship to practice.

However, it is a corrective to the naive scientism of much social research and is an approach which challenges given definitions of problems.

Essentially it is a research style which can be called 'ideology critique' in its attempt to treat critically taken-for-granted assumptions and definitions and to place ideas in relation to their class origins. The final report of the Coventry Community Development Project[10] is an example of this mode. Another is in 'Neighbourhood Politics and Housing Opportunities,[11] which seeks to uncover some of the 'hidden' purposes of a housing queue and points system and to relate how commonly held ideas about the rightness and fairness of such a system derive, not naturally or by chance, but from the way housing is administered – from the social relations underlying housing allocation.

For community workers, I would argue, research as ideology critique and the procedures of that process are essential to the worker as research consumer in order to be able to place and interpret, and so criticise positively, plans, proposals and ideas for the neighbourhood in which he works so that he can say in whose interest such proposals are made.

If this seems unrelated to what has gone before I would refer the reader to a most telling article by Peter Marris. He writes in the context of the disillusion and failure which has beset a lot of community development work (especially in America). His comments should be studied by those interested in developing a strong research and evaluation element to community work practice in Britain. Essentially he writes about the difficulty of applying scientific research methods to social enquiry. He concludes that we need to conceive of community action and development programmes as explorations of 'the adaptability of our social institutions'. In this light 'research into community action is contemporary political history' and its components are 'to be everywhere, know everything that happened and how it happened, to record all this – and then, behind the mass of details and the accidents of personality to discern the general pattern of issues which determined these events'.[12]

The methods and styles and approaches of conventional social research can help in this task with their proposals for organising and planning the implicit quest for omniscience and, most important of all, with their stress on clear, careful, assiduous recording. Research methods, however, will not provide the crucial answers, for as Marris reminds us:

'From the perspective of differing ideologies and interests the same history reveals different patterns, which are all insights into its meaning, though their implications may be contradictory. Hence the researcher has to decide for whose interests he speaks, and whom he is seeking to influence, while still recognising that the force of his argument depends on the intellectual integrity of his analysis not his commitment.'

Likewise the community worker; but in addition the effects of research will be a challenge to his intellectual integrity and to his commitment.

That, in short, is the essential contribution of research to the knowledge and skills of the community worker.

NOTES AND REFERENCES

1 '. . . careful search or enquiry *after or for*; endeavour to discover facts by scientific study of a subject, course of critical investigation . . .' *Concise Oxford Dictionary* (London, Oxford University Press, 1951), p. 1038.

2 *Current Issues in Community Work* (London, Routledge & Kegan Paul, 1973), ch. 5.

3 Bob Ashcroft and Keith Jackson, 'Adult Education and Social Action', in D. Jones and M. Mayo (eds), *Community Work One* (London, Routledge & Kegan Paul, 1974), pp. 44-65.

4 See 'The Sparkbrook West Story', *West Midlands Grassroots No. 12*, April 1974.

5 *Workers on the Scrapheap* (A report for the Birmingham Community Development Project, 1975).

6 See Further Reading below. Chapter 2 of Worsley, *Introducing Sociology* is particularly helpful.

7 On participant observation the following will be useful: (a) C. Sellitz, M. Jahoda, M. Deutscke and G. W. Cook, *Research Methods in Social Relations* (Methuen, 1965); (b) W. Filstead (ed.), *Qualitative Methodology and Theory* (Markham, 1970); (c) Howard S. Becker, 'Inference and Proof in Participant Observation', *American Sociological Review*, 23rd June, 1958.

8 Some examples (not including the census) are: The Registrar General, *Statistical Reviews, Quarterly Reviews*, and *Annual Reports*; Dept of Education, *Statistics of Education*; Dept of the Environment, quarterly and annual *Local Housing Statistics*; Institute of Municipal Treasurers and Accountants (IMTA), *Housing Statistics* and *Housing Rent Statistics*; Dept of Health and Social Security, *On the State of the Public Health* and *Annual Statistical Report*. General Registrar Office, *Studies on Medical and Population Subjects*.

9 Counter Information Services, 54 Shaftesbury Avenue, London W1; *Community Action*, P.O. Box 665, London SW1X 8DZ.

10 *Coventry and Hillfields: Prosperity and the Persistence of Inequality* (CDP, Coventry, Final Report, March 1975).

11 J. Lambert, B. Blackaby and C. Paris, 'Neighbourhood Politics and Housing Opportunities', *Community Development Journal 10* (2nd April, 1975).

12 P. Marris, 'Experimenting in Social Reform', in Jones and Mayo (eds), op. cit., pp. 245-59.

FURTHER READING

P. Worsley, *Introducing Sociology* (Penguin Books, 1970), ch. 2.

M. Stacey, *Methods of Social Research* (Pergamon, 1969).

G. Easthope, *History of Social Research Methods* (Longman, 1974).

W. Goode and P. Hatt, *Methods in Social Research* (McGraw Hill, 1952).

C. Sellitz, M. Jahoda, M. Deutscke and G. W. Cook, *Research Methods in Social Relations* (Methuen, 1965).

C. Moser and G. Kalton, *Survey Methods in Social Investigation* (Heinemann Educational, 1972).

S. A. Richardson *et al.*, *Interviewing: Its Forms and Functions* (Basic Books, 1965).

W. Filstead (ed.), *Qualitative Methodology and Theory* (Markham, 1970).

A. Vidich, J. Bensman, and M. Stein, *Reflections on Community Studies* (Harper, 1972).

Chapter 8

MANAGEMENT, PLANNING AND COMMUNITY WORK

Jimmy Algie, Clive Miller and Norman Kam

Community workers traditionally see management as what hierarchic bosses do (when formally commanding 'subordinates' to perform certain duties), what supervisors and overseers do (when watching over employees' shoulders to monitor their every move), what bureaucratic officials do (when obsessively processing forms), and as what consumers confront when they 'apply for' services. Management is imagined to be about acquiring high-powered leadership qualities, making dramatic snap-of-the-fingers judgements after momentary reflection, handling tricky staff relations, manipulating personnel into doing unpleasant things with pep talks or threats of dismissal, instituting mechanical office routines, and establishing accountancy devices to check office costs, staff numbers and time keeping. 'Manager', 'organisation', 'control', 'hierarchy', and 'system' are words that raise the community worker's hackles, and recur throughout management studies.

At first glance, management studies seem at odds with everything community workers are about. This is reinforced by bitter experiences with some grey-suited functionaries in government bureaucracies and conformist, elitist, manipulative overtones of old-style management literature.

Yet community workers recognise that they have somehow to manage their activities. Managing is essentially about evolving decisions in the light of relevant values and information from all participants involved. It is about groups working effectively according to agreed choices. Community workers jointly set and agree objectives for action with others. They mobilise and allocate scarce human, physical, financial resources. They co-ordinate and take part in various operations, and seek to generate change. They acquire, use and communicate relevant information, seeking to adapt their working style to each situation confronted. They participate in structuring role and interagency relations. They evaluate effects of their own and others' actions.

Most community workers realise they are involved in these processes, which are the subject matter of management studies, and discuss them constantly. This is not surprising: community work activities involve managing, planning and organising situations in order to achieve desired changes in co-operation with others and to avoid chaos. Instead of painstakingly, haphazardly learning from trial and error, community workers (and their clientele) might well benefit were they to use, critically and cautiously, some management and planning approaches to working effectively.

We shall now endeavour to make some relevant connections between management studies and community work, using a framework (Figure 8.1) which community workers have often found helpful in managing their work systematically.

The first stage is to consider alternative possible *values and objectives* community groups might seek to realise in action. Community workers specify these in terms of particular *social needs and problems* and in terms of particular *community work activities* designed to make some impact on the needs confronted. The objectives chosen vary according to which *interest groups* influence and are influenced by the community groups concerned, and what objectives and values these interest groups themselves subscribe to.

In addition to choosing between alternative objectives, community groups have to choose between alternative *strategies* they might adopt in attempting to achieve their chosen objectives. Each strategy implies different *roles* for the community worker, thence a different range of *skills*.

In evolving a systematic basis for working, community groups clearly have significant choices to make at different levels of planning and action. These choices may be aided by analysing alternative possible *criteria* (which might inform such choices) and the various *kinds of environment* in which the community work group is concerned (and which might influence choices). Various community work and management *technologies and methods* become relevant in carrying out whatever community work action is required, given the objectives, strategies and roles agreed. Evaluating *results* of community work action against the objectives originally formulated provides the basis for revising and developing subsequent action. We shall explore this framework further, indicating and exemplifying the kind of contribution management studies might make to community work in the areas of setting objectives, ranking criteria for policy choice, and developing community work strategies, with their associated roles. We shall also examine some management technologies and concepts that may help community workers better to understand and intervene in the communities and organisations with which they are concerned.

SETTING OF OBJECTIVES

Two methods increasingly used are management by objectives (MBO)

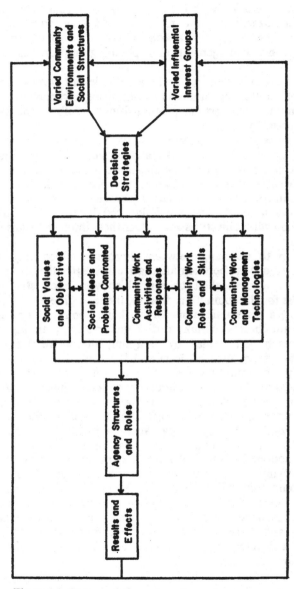

Figure 8.1 *Framework for community work management*

expounded by Humble[1] and Reddin[2]; and planning, programming, budgeting systems (PPBS), expounded by Novick.[3] These focused management studies on what outcomes, results or benefits were produced by services and the value implications of different modes of work, rather than merely upon mechanics of efficient service delivery. The aims were to render agency and staff objectives more explicit, review pros and cons of alternatives, tailor services to achieve these objectives, and evaluate results of service delivery against agreed objectives. These methods have been developed through more sophisticated approaches. 'Priority scaling' and 'integrated management, planning and action systems' (IMPACTS, for short) usher in open-ended participative and questioning approaches to value issues more relevant for community workers than traditional procedures.

Priority Scaling
Priority scaling is a systematic method by which agency staff and consumer representatives may jointly set desired priorities, given scarce agency resources available for allocation. Allocation choices are made as between which specific social needs and problems the agency shall respond to, and at what level of service. The diverse choices of staff and consumers are integrated into an agreed, coherent agency policy on priorities. This is done by analysing the value implications of the choices, interlinking common elements in each set of choices, and then forging agreements using various scaling and decision methods. This policy is implemented through a systematic programme of change by which existing agency priorities are replaced by the newly agreed priorities at every working level, from overall agency budgeting to specific caseload management. The results are tested and revised according to agreed criteria for effectiveness.

IMPACTS
The integrated, management, planning and action systems approach (IMPACTS) is related to priority scaling. Here, specific targets and activities of front-line workers are reviewed to determine the wider value implications involved. Simultaneously, statements of overall agency policies and plans are reviewed in terms of how they might be translated into agency practice and action. The stated policies are compared with those implied by agency practice. Conversely, practice is compared with action implied by stated agency policies.

The resulting mismatch between stated and actual situations provides a basis for questioning and devising alternative agency plans and action in terms of what is desirable and feasible. As many staff and consumer representatives as possible are involved in decisions on both the value and action issues, and an integrated programme of policy and action is thereby derived for the agency.

Both approaches are partially exemplified below, and more fully elsewhere by Algie.[4] They open up value issues and action opportunities within social services agencies of a kind community workers are constantly calling for. They have direct application as methods for determining current and desired objectives of communities and their members, underlying values implicit in how everyday community life is run and in the aspirations of community members. They each require that certain things are made more explicit: the actual and implicit priority accorded to various social needs, their treatment in terms of time and effort expended on various community activities, how resources are distributed, and what changes are required if desired community values, objectives and priorities are to be fulfilled. This analysis then becomes the basis for agency planning so that genuinely client-based, needs-based services are developed.

The work of Uhlig[5] and Baier and Rescher[6] has indicated how these methods may be applied on a community-wide basis in the American situation. Few, if any, British applications have been documented, though the literature and practice of British community work is permeated by issues of determining, deciding and developing community values, objectives, priorities and action.

In selecting objectives and action strategies, community workers are inevitably attempting to sort out, in some manner, the conflicting values and objectives of interest groups. They map varied sources of community influence in some form. They are concerned with reviewing the net effects made on the community situation by the various influences acting simultaneously or over time. They have to evolve viable responses to the situation produced by these contrasting influences, and community workers themselves function as an interest group whose values and persuasions influence community conditions.

The interest groups with which community workers are concerned include central government departments, local authority councillors and officers, pressure groups, profit-making organisations, consumers, local residents, and neighbourhood professionals such as doctors and teachers. Any list of interest groups is shorthand for displaying the varied community perceptions operative when major social decisions are taken.

Community workers often have to analyse objectives and operating methods of relevant interest groups. These objectives are rarely explicit. Community workers need to get behind overt policy and public relations statements to uncover policies implicit in how interest groups act in practice. So-called 'technical' decisions (from magistrates' sentencing practices to land use planning procedures) often amount to major policy statements with wide-ranging community ramifications. Understanding how interest groups distinguish between technical (or 'non-problematic') and policy (or 'problematic') areas of activity is critical in interpreting and influencing their behaviour, as ethnomethodologists frequently demonstrate.[7] Simulation gaming has proved a particularly helpful management tool for community workers in understanding the effects of varied interest groups in community decision making and evolving effective responses.[8] What do all the conflicting interests and objectives add up to for the community? How can the community worker find some way through the mesh of objectives and interests so that the community as a whole gains rather than loses? Though themselves one interest group among many, community workers operate as catalysts seeking to find viable, effective paths through the push and pull of conflicting community interest groups. In handling their dual role, community workers have to consider alternative criteria by which social policies and plans for the community may be determined. An outline list of such criteria for policy choice is now given.

ALTERNATIVE POLICY CRITERIA

Choices have to be made between what degrees of priority will be given to the following criteria. By ranking the criteria, community workers may develop a coherent basis for which policies they shall pursue and how they would wish the resources of their own and other agencies to be allocated accordingly.

Preventability
How far shall we concentrate resources and attention on those social problems which are potentially preventable?

Severity
How far should we allocate resources to 'severest' forms of social impediment or distress irrespective of our current capability of effecting major change?

Agency Capability
How far shall we attend only to those social situations where we can potentially effect greatest change?

Resource Availability
To what extent shall we develop services in accordance with resources already available, irrespective of manifest or latent community needs?

Ramification
To what extent shall we concentrate on problems having the widest ranging community impact and ramifying effects on others rather than self-contained problems?

Prevalence
Shall we provide resources in direct proportion to the prevalence of community problems? Shall the largest problems, as defined by numbers affected, attract most resources?

Degree of Emergency
To what extent shall we respond to immediate crises or emergencies as felt by clients?

Unmet Needs
Should most resources be applied to previously unmet or unrecognised needs, or to those which will remain unmet unless we tackle them ourselves, irrespective of existing skills, interests, knowledge and resources?

Clientele Selectivity
How far will we focus resources on some specific client groups to the exclusion of others, irrespective of demands on service?

Geographical Selectivity
How far will we focus resources on geographically defined areas of greatest need (e.g. depressed zone's, educational priority areas) to the exclusion of a more territorially even spread of services?

Base of Administration
Are we going to allocate most resources to what we are most efficient at (e.g. to what is administratively easiest to run)?

Diagnostic Focus
Do we want to spend most of our energies on expert diagnosis of problems which are then referred to other agencies for treatment?

Treatment Focus
Shall we invest maximum resources in enlarging our capacity to treat problems as referred and prediagnosed by others?

Advocacy Focus
How far should our major efforts be geared to inducing changes in neighbouring agency policies?

Distribution of Interest
How far shall we allocate our resources in response to the varying degrees of influence of different interest groups upon us?

Such criteria are relevant not only in the community group's decisions about its policies but also in clarifying and influencing the policies used by service agencies. Given the catalyst role many community workers seek to perform, it behoves them to be clearer than most as to their comparative weighting of the criteria and how these may be reflected in service delivery decisions. Operational methods by which community workers might assign comparative values and weightings as between such criteria are detailed elsewhere by Algie.[9]

<h2 style="text-align:center">COMMUNITY WORK STRATEGIES</h2>

A key question running through the choice of community work strategies appears to be: who is seen as the prime mover in mobilising (as distinct from providing) community services?

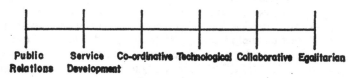

Figure 8.2 *Community Work Strategies*

At the end of the spectrum, the worker's employing agency is seen as prime mover. This 'public relations' strategy emphasises 'selling' certain services to the community. At the other end of the continuum, the community itself is seen as prime mover. Here the 'egalitarian strategy emphasises major shifts in the community power structure as basic to improving community services. The continuum of strategies is outlined below, together with implications for community worker roles.

Public Relations Strategy
This focuses on improving agency methods in presenting and communicating their policies and services to community 'publics' and interest groups. In the narrowest sense, the agency uses the community worker to improve its image in the community, to pacify certain vociferous and discontented community groups, gain more agency resources informally by communicating persuasively to volunteers, and help the agency prepare its case in forthcoming disputes. Conflict between agency and community is kept in a low key. Any service changes proposed are not expected to require major change in agency structures.

Community workers adopting this strategy establish a network of links with several community groups, disseminate selected information about the agency to its community, ensure that agency policies are well represented to significant groups and that the agency is kept informed of community attitudes towards its services. Without underestimating the problems and needs of communicating information, many community workers object strongly to being used instrumentally in this public relations role.

In a wider sense, the strategy involves community workers in alerting potential consumers to their rights and providing adequate access to services. Consumers may find it a mammoth task to negotiate the maze of welfare rights and discover particular services. The agency may not be aware overall of how its priorities policies, say, in the form of eligibility rules, is actually functioning and perceived by consumers. The appearance and location of agency facilities may discourage client use, thus decreasing community take-up of services. This may lead to the community worker adopting the role of consumer informant, also charged with monitoring and providing feedback on consumer attitudes and perceptions through ongoing consumer surveys.

Guiding consumers and service providers through the maze of eligibility rules or alternative services provides the community worker with a major headache. Algorithms help here. These are simply display devices that take client or service provider through a series of straightforward questions structured to produce YES/NO answers. Questions may focus on decisions as to which legislation (hence which services) apply in particular client situations, and agreed service delivery procedures.[10] Algorithms are one of many aids relevant in this type of role drawn from branches of management studies concerned with public relations,[11] communications[12][13] and information science.[14]

Service Development Strategy

This strategy focuses on improving and developing specific services, getting services more effectively delivered to people needing them, and linking potential consumers with service providers. Feedback from community members to service producers is used to correct and develop services so they become responsive to changing community needs, interest and values. Stress is placed on reorganising services, taking into account current findings on service effectiveness. The service development strategy marks the first point on the continuum of strategies where agency restructuring may become an explicit objective, which is mirrored in the stress on action objectives to ensure feedback and change.

Community workers operating in the service development role have direct face-to-face interaction with service consumers, with neighbourhood residents, with citizens sharing common problems, interests or objectives, and with service providers and other decision makers who influence community objectives. Service development is a matter of co-ordinating the work of all these groups so that agency services can be redesigned to provide a better match with community needs. Systems developed in management studies for designing new services[15] have enormous potential for community workers adopting this strategy.

Co-ordinative Strategy

Co-ordinative objectives may involve community workers in what has come to be called community organisation. Neighbouring services and service professionals (general practitioners, teachers, housing managers, clergy, etc.) are mobilised on behalf of social services objectives. The requirement that services be co-ordinated reflects the view that social needs and problems are interrelated and changing whether at the level of the individual or the level of society. Co-ordination problems increasingly arise between intra-organisational divisions as the organisation becomes more comprehensive, interorganisationally and interprofessionally, as agencies become more specialised. The problems relate to differences in types of clientele, service, specialism, geographical and hierarchic division. Co-ordination involves systematically bringing segmented services into an effective, coherent system. Management work organisation analysis[16][17] in merger theory[18] and in systems modelling[19] is relevant here.

Technological Strategy

Using the technological strategy, certain resources (including knowledge and information) are placed at the disposal of community groups to use as they choose. This strategy is perhaps summarised in the community development approach. This aims to stimulate increased community responsibility for services and for people in need, and to encourage self-help, self-direction and mutual aid by community members. The expected overall effect is to unite community members' own efforts with those of public agencies in improving social, cultural and economic conditions in their communities, supported by on-tap technical and professional resources.

This strategy emphasises community self-help and attempts to change the community power structure. It implies that the community worker place himself in the role of *professional adviser* or *expert consultant*. He provides professional information, advice and skills to community groups on how they might achieve their objectives. His advice may cover such matters as collecting reliable data on community problems and attitudes, methods of searching out and locating certain individuals in need, planning sequences of action to achieve ends, devising means of evaluating the effectiveness of services *vis-à-vis* social problems they are designed to handle, developing strategies for mobilising power in support of certain courses of action, and improving communication channels and structures accordingly. The relevant management literature in this area is vast and potentially the most helpful of all, if it could only be translated into language accessible to community workers.

Collaborative Strategy

The theme of some community work revolves around community participation. Interest groups of all kinds are helped to participate in formulating and deciding any significant community decision and action as far as is feasible. Developing more democratic, participative systems for community decision making becomes central. The objective is to derive social and psychological benefits resulting from participation, strengthening collaborative and integrative attitudes, and group problems-solving capabilities and group development in the community at large. This approach, often referred to by the term 'community integration', implies that participation of diverse interest groups in decision making is of value in its own right, almost irrespective of the specific outcomes produced, so long as various groups learn to work more effectively together.

The collaborative strategy implies the community worker's role is that of *co-ordinator, reconciler or go-between*. The community worker is concerned with analysing diverse values and objectives, co-ordinating diverse activities of different groups, structuring interagency and intergroup mechanisms by which fruitful exchanges may occur, and helping resolution of conflicts which impede relevant action. Much work has been achieved in the management studies field which suggest how, specifically and practically, such participative systems may be achieved.[20]

Egalitarian Strategy

The primary focus of the egalitarian strategy is on gaining redistribution of power, resources and opportunities among community groups. This involves the worker in community and organisational politics, frequently leading to social action and confrontation with those who use their power and resources to impede the equalisation process. The objective is to enable or stimulate collective social action on significant issues by working in an *advocacy role* on behalf of underprivileged groups so they may protect and realise their own interests more fully. This may mean using established channels, negotiating, using pressure, or, in the extreme, protest activities such as picketing, marches, demonstrations, sit-ins and strikes. Unlike the collaborative strategy, which also demands political skills, structural change in all the target systems is here seen as primary. The Alinksy-style *social activist* role, sometimes providing a built-in (even paid) opposition to the agency system, is implied by the extreme form of this strategy.

In respect of the egalitarian strategy, the areas in which management studies have most to offer include, firstly, the analysis of power and of the distributive economic effects of alternative policies, to which Niskanen[21] provides a useful introduction; and, secondly, the politics of decision making[22][23] and some of the work on conflict in and between organisations.[24]

Strategies and Roles

Discrepancies in possible strategies and roles of the community worker are familiar in social services agencies. They reflect varied values and objectives pursued by those who sanctioned the community work role at the outset. The effective worker has to negotiate an appropriate balance of alternative objectives and roles, depending on the community and agency situations concerned. As his objectives and roles vary, so will the kind of action he takes. This position is by no means as pragmatic as it may sound, for it may demand continuous radical adjustments not only by the worker in respect of his mode of practice but also by the community groups with which he is concerned and by his employing agency. For example, if the employing agency is hierarchically organised a more or less fixed structure of roles and associated duties holds. The effective community worker by contrast is one whose role will be continuously changing depending on (among other things) the stage of community development currently attained. This implies a more polyarchic form of structuring for the employing organisation (as discussed later) wherein role changes are the order of the day.[25] Recognising this, many community workers have sought employment outside of public service bureaucracies which seem irredeemably hierarchic in structure and mode of operation. However, this neglects the contribution that the presence of community workers within public service hierarchies may make to developing less hierarchic forms of structure.

Management studies are essentially concerned with methods of matching the highly varied alternative interests, objectives, services, methods and roles involved in complex situations of the kind here analysed in respect of community work, so that action involved gains some coherence and relevance to real life. This inevitably leads to specifying community work objectives farther, usually in terms of specific social conditions. For all community workers, whatever role they adopt, are ultimately concerned with meeting some specific community needs, resolving some specific social problems or reducing certain disabling social conditions. From this perspective, all community workers function as change agents. In this role, the community worker may find management studies related to engineering change in the face of resistance increasingly relevant.[26]

TECHNOLOGY OF COMMUNITY WORK

Depending on which objectives and activities the community worker selects, the skills required to pursue these objectives and undertake these activities in an effective manner vary. Skills analysis becomes relevant at this point.[27]

Specific skills are usually based on certain technologies or methodologies for handling problems. Community workers are usually seeking to get to grips with a complex range of social variables interacting one with another and changing dynamically over time and summarised in the term 'community'. They usually have minimal information available to them, and

E

this renders their decisions highly risky and uncertain. This is reinforced in that the effects of most of these decisions and operations can only be judged over a relatively long time-span. Management studies are concerned with just these problems of uncertainty, variety, complexity, changeableness and risk, as is well exemplified by Beer.[28]

Taking one of the many management approaches to handling such problems, let us briefly explore the potential use of simulation models for community work purposes. The community is seen as a system. It has some degree of coherence, pattern and directionality, despite the apparent randomness and variety of divergent needs, interests and purposes of the manifold individuals and groups comprising the community concerned. A community, in the sense of the smallest territorial group based on a geographical locality that can embrace all aspects of life, still has meaning in villages, small towns, long established neighbourhoods and for certain people like the aged, the very young, the single mother with a young family. Modern communities cannot usually be understood in terms of themselves alone. Each segment may be more closely linked with similar segments in other communities than with dissimilar segments in the same community. People in modern communities often have more in common with others having the same work, social and cultural interest than with their neighbours. For many, membership of various communities of interests and association unrelated to geographical propinquity is more significant than neighbourhood locality. Within any area, there are groups, networks and communities of interest who interconnect in various ways and to varying degrees, and who occupy overlapping territories. The community worker is also concerned with non-place communities. He works with systems or networks of interrelated individuals, families, groups, organisations and interests defined in terms of the needs, interests or objectives at issue and tasks to be undertaken. When these are added together certain patterns result. These patterns are mapped in simulation models of the community as a system.

Simulation Modelling

Simulation models are essentially simplified maps of complex situations, as London Transport maps chart the complex underground train system or architect's plans prefigure complex buildings. Dynamic situations may also be simulated, as with the highway engineer's model of traffic flows through a city. Using the aid of competent systems analysts, models of the community situation may be developed for each community with which the community worker is concerned. Thus, Systems Simulation Ltd developed computerised models of how various social problems develop within a community and the effect of agency interrelations on these problems.[29] Forrester[30] and Meadows[31] developed more general models of community functioning.

These models may be used to predict likely developments of community problems. Where accurate information about some variables is unavailable, intelligent estimates are made. To the extent that the predictions arranged by the models are accurate, the models may be taken as more or less accurate (though inevitably simplified) representations of the community situation. To the extent that predictions are inaccurate, the models may be 'tuned' by varying the relationship between relevant variables until principles on which they are built more accurately reflect the actual situation. More specific information may be gathered through community surveys and research studies.

Once predictive accuracy is achieved, the simulation model may be said to reflect community reality. At this point, the effect of various possible interventions in the community situation by community workers may be tested in advance of risky and dangerous 'suck-it-and-see' experiments with the real-life situation. Moreover, empirical research surveys may be more precisely targeted on specific hypotheses about the community on which decision makers require some answer, given that the simulation model can be used to point the way.

Major problems arise directly any technological development is proposed to community workers, especially anything involving computer hardware. They have first-hand experience of the ill effects of so many technological experiments in communities and individuals they serve, and are justifiably sceptical. They have seen the ill effects of slum-clearance schemes, new town developments, high-rise flats built by people called 'systems engineers', computerised information systems and so on, all of which have intruded on individual privacy and produced mechanistic procedures which hit the poorest hardest. Roszak[32] and Illich[33] state the arguments persuasively.

The suggestion here made is that some of the new technologies may be harnessed for other objectives than those for which they have been customarily used. They may be used on the consumer's behalf as well as on behalf of bureaucratic authorities. They may be used to produce consumer benefits as well as disbenefits, provided social factors are taken into full account. They may be used to achieve less bureaucratic and more open modes of organisation without producing chaos.[34] For this purpose, it is vital that the contributions and perceptions of community workers be used. More important, it is vital that community-responsive groups (including community workers) gain control, to some degree, of how such technologies are used.

A simulation model may be used by an autocratic group to gain greater control over its community or by a community to direct its own development. Either way, both groups require information about the community situation overall, not merely segmented and partitioned information about some artificially delimited aspect of community life of the kind provided by the bureaucracies involved. To the extent that access to results of management and planning technologies are equally open to all participants involved, their development is to be encouraged. To the extent that the results are owned by elites and bureaucrats, their development is justifiably deplored.

Rejection of potentially increased knowledge and understanding is undesirable on all counts, provided that all parties have equal access to developing knowledge and equal power over its use. One of the community worker's many functions is to ensure that such increased knowledge is not developed for the benefit of privileged groups at the expense of the under-privileged, or that it is inaccessible to all but the already powerful. It is presumably not the function of community workers to suppress knowledge and information. Given that confidentiality safeguards are required in respect of many specific bits of information associated with individual members of the community, this can technically be arranged with greater security when systematic information systems are used. The major requirement is that the rules as to who does not get what information and limits on how each piece of information is to be used are agreed and estab-lished at the outset. The community worker has a vital role to perform in gaining agreement on appropriate safeguards in this area.

ORGANISATION AND SOCIAL STRUCTURES

This systems approach to the community situation implies a radically new conception of social and organisational structures. Many community workers oppose the existing forms of hierarchically organised bureaucratic structure which they daily have to handle. Their opposition may rest on grounds of value (e.g. a belief in democratic decision making at all levels and stages) or of effectiveness (e.g. hierarchically organised local authority departments frequently seem ineffectual and inadaptive to community needs). If they turn to traditional organisational theory, workers confront a set of apologies for organisational hierarchy,[35] just as they confront apologies for social hierarchies in traditional sociological literature.[36]

Fortunately, new developments in organisation studies (which ally with sociological developments) are based on clearer recognition of serious problems endemic in hierarchic structures of organisations and communities. A summary of these alternative approaches is provided elsewhere.[37] These alternatives concern the development of more demo-cratic, egalitarian, adaptive, open and socially planned systems of organisa-tion, together with structures which may provide more effective responses to community problems confronted. The ethos, values and methods embraced by these new forms of organisation structure commonly referred to as 'polyarchy' seem to accord more with the beliefs and methods common among community workers than traditional hierarchic approaches to organisational and social structures. The hierarchic approach to organisations and communities is a matter of ranked and sectionalised authority divisions among positions which are formally institutionalised. This leads in turn to a set of working and social relations which are based on lineal relations between 'superiors' and 'subordinates' in organisational hierarchies, between leaders and led ('haves' and 'have-nots') in social structures.

The specific bureaucratic relations involved in social services departmental organisations have been clearly explained by Rowbottom et al.[38] The social relations involved have been documented by Victorian anthropologists when analysing primitive tribes from a traditionalist Western perspective.[39]

The polyarchic approach to structuring organisations and communities is a matter of democratically, participatively evolving decisions and action. Polyarchic structures are built around objectives mutually agreed by all involved and flexibly adjusted to changing patterns of activity. They take the form of multiple, overlapping systems of co-operation in which each group simultaneously generates and checks the work of each other group. New types of role relation are involved in which no person is 'subordinated' to another, responsibility for decisions being vested directly in the person taking the action, rather than in his boss or overseer. The specific relations involved are explained elsewhere in terms of social services agencies.[40] The social relations involved have been documented by modern anthropologists when analysing social structures from a polyarchic perspective.[41] Developments in organisational studies have illuminated new ways of investigating and analysing both agency and social structures. Community workers cannot afford to neglect these developments.

CONCLUSION

It is clear that effective community work involves managing, planning and organising skills of a high order. Many community workers have developed these skills through the trials and errors of experience. The potential use of management and planning studies for community workers lies in the development in systematic approaches and methods for handling many of the problems they daily encounter. They are also of value in helping the community worker match his choices of alternative objectives, strategies, methods and roles so that they form some coherent system of action, and thus a basis for evaluating effectiveness of his action. Ultimately, this evaluation involves assessing the overall impact on the community situation of service activities of various agencies including the impact of community work services.

REFERENCES

1 J. Humble, *Improving Business Results* (Maidenhead, McGraw Hill, 1968).
2 W. Reddin, *Effective MBO* (London Management Publications, 1971).
3 D. Novick (ed.), *Program Budgeting* (Harvard University Press, 1967).
4 J. Algie, *Social Values, Objectives and Action* (London, Kogan Page, 1975) and Comment, '*Social Work Today*', 6, No. 11, August 1975.
5 R. Uhlig, *A Study in Social Service Values and Priorities* (Pittsburg Health and Welfare Council, 1956).
6 K. Baier and N. Rescher (eds), *Values and the Future* (Ontario, The Free Press, 1969).
7 H. Garfinkel, *Studies in Ethnomethodology* (New Jersey, Prentice-Hall, 1967).
8 A. S. Hall and J. Algie, *A Management Game for the Social Services* (London, Bedford Square Press, 1974).
9 J. Algie, *Social Values, Objectives and Action* (London, Kogan Page, 1975).
10 J. Algie and C. Miller, *Skills in Social Services* (London, Kogan Page, 1976).
11 H. Stephenson, *Handbook of Public Relations* (New York, McGraw-Hill, 1960).
12 L. Thayer, *Communication and Communication Systems* (Homewood, Illinois, R. D. Irwin, 1968).
13 W. Haney, *Communication and Organizational Behaviour: Text and Cases* (Homewood, Illinois, R. D. Irwin, 1973).
14 A. McDonough, *Information Economics and Management Systems* (New York, McGraw-Hill, 1963).
15 E. A. Pessemier, *New Product Decisions* (New York, McGraw-Hill, 1966).
16 N. Evan, 'The Organisational Set: Towards a Theory of Interorganisational Relations', in J. Thompson (ed.), *Approaches to Organisation Design* (University of Pittsburg Press, 1966).
17 S. Levine, P. White and B. Paul, 'Community Interorganizational Problems of Providing Medical Care and Social Services', *American Journal of Public Health*, 53, August 1963.
18 J. Algie, *New Approaches to Organising* (London, Kogan Page, 1976).
19 S. Beer, *The Brain of the Firm* (Allen Lane The Penguin Press, 1972).
20 J. Algie, *New Approaches to Organising*, op. cit.
21 W. A. Niskanen, *Bureaucracy and Representative Government* (Chicago, Aldine-Atherton, 1971).
22 A. Wildavsky, 'The Self-evaluating Organisation', *Public Administration Review*, 32, 1972.
23 D. Braybrooke and C. E. Lindblom, *A Strategy of Decision* (New York, Free Press, 1970).
24 L. Pondy, 'Organisational Conflict: Concepts and Models', *Administrative Science Quarterly*, XII, September 1967.
25 J. Algie, '*Social Work Today*', 6, No. 11, August 1975.
26 N. Gross, J. B. Giacquinta and M. Bernstein, *Implementing Organisational Innovations* (New York, Harper Row, 1971).
27 J. Algie and C. Miller, *Skills in Social Services* (London, Kogan Page, 1976).
28 S. Beer, *Decision and Control* (London, Wiley, 1966).
29 J. Algie, 'The Technology of Social Work', *Spectator*, London, 22nd July, 1972.

30 J. Forrester, *Urban Dynamics* (MIT Press, Cambridge, Mass, 1969).
31 D. L. Meadows *et al.*, *Limits to Growth* (Washington, Potomac Assoc. Inc., 1972).
32 T. Rozak, *Where the Wasteland Ends: Politics and Transcendence in Post Industrial Society* (London, Faber & Faber, 1974).
33 I. Illich, *Celebration of Awareness* (Middlesex, Penguin, 1969).
34 See, for instance, S. Beer, *Platform for Change* (London, Wiley, 1975) and J. Algie, *New Approaches to Organising* (London, Kogan Page, 1976).
35 R. Rowbottom *et al.*, *Social Services Departments. Developing patterns of work and organisation* (London, Heinemann, 1974).
36 T. Parsons, *The Structure of Social Action* (London, McGraw-Hill, 1937).
37 See J. Algie, Comment, *Social Work Today*, 21st August, 1975 and *New Approaches to Organising* (London, Kogan Page, 1976).
38 R. Rowbottom *et al.*, op. cit.
39 A. R. Radcliffe-Brown and D. Forde (eds), *African Systems of Kinship and Marriage* (Oxford University Press, 1950).
40 J. Algie, Comment, *Social Work Today*, op. cit. and *New Approaches to Organising*, op. cit.
41 J. Boissevain, *Friends of Friends* (Oxford, Basil Blackwell, 1974).

Chapter 9

LINKING LEARNING TO EXPERIENCE IN COMMUNITY WORK TRAINING

Nicholas Derricourt

The purpose of this chapter is not to catalogue the knowledge and skills of community workers but to indicate that these may be developed within a model of learning that I call the 'direct experience' model. This is an inclusive, non-elitist pattern of education which provides opportunities for training in community work to both outside professionals and community residents. Its methods of study are rooted within the field and life experiences of the students.

The first Gulbenkian report[1] offered a three-part synthesis of the varieties of community work which provides as helpful a start as anywhere for a consideration of the training of community workers:

direct work with local people in the form of a community development service;
facilitating agency and interagency co-ordination and sustaining and promoting organised groups;
community planning and policy formulation.

A criticism of these categories has been sharply put by Naish and Filkin:

'The Gulbenkian report also failed to *indicate priorities of work* and a community worker will need to get clear that work in any of these spheres should be geared to the primary activity of working for resource redistribution into deprived areas (redistribution of resources involves the redistribution of material goods, cash, services, information, emotional resources, power, etc.).'[2]

The references to the 'primary activity' of community work, the broad range of resources, and the reminder that 'deprived areas' are the location of many community work tasks, suggest that Gulbenkian's three categories of community work need to be understood in the light of particular priorities. These in turn give rise to a need for workers with a particular sort of training. From this suggestion follows some important implications:

1 Training must enable students to gain an understanding both of the locality in which work is to occur and of the institutions which currently control and manage resource distribution.

2 The requisite skills and techniques follow from the need for effective organising of groups for the purposes of resource distribution.

3 Local people who are members and leaders of such groups are as much community workers as professional or outside organisers, and are therefore part of the student* population for whom courses of community work training should be prepared.

I would argue that most institutions putting on courses in community work are traditionally geared to provide only for those outsiders, professionals and non-residents, who get involved in community work. Moreover, few institutions have as teachers those who have direct and successful experience of this sort of community work. Furthermore, whatever skills a teaching institution may have in providing students with a working model of a resource-distributing power structure, or however good it is at explaining and simulating small group organisational practice, it must have only very limited and necessarily elitist capacity to instruct its predominantly middle-class students about what life is like in working-class deprived areas of modern cities.

For courses to become accessible to a wide audience and for them to be made effective both for the paid and unpaid, middle class and working class, professional and non-professional, male and female, young and old, they must avoid exclusive and elitist forms. And for a course to direct itself to the primary activity of resource distribution to deprived areas, then it must be firmly anchored in the concrete experience of inhabitants of working-class localities and in an analysis of the institutional controls on existing resource distribution. So, although there are specific skills and techniques which community workers need, there is an essential task for courses: to draw out and build up the experience which will enable students to discover the orientation and perspective within which community work is to occur. What qualifies people for community work of this sort is a kind of involvement; their direct experience at work or in life provides the material, the base on which skills and knowledge for community work may be developed.

With this by way of introduction, I will now look at some specific areas in which to expand and elucidate how this style of community work

* Although I normally prefer the term 'course members' to 'students', the latter will be used in the chapter to avoid confusion with councillors. It is an inappropriate term to use in this chapter, because it conveys an impression which undermines my argument that more people should be included in community work training than those usually conjured up by the term 'student'. The term 'teacher' is used throughout with similar reservations.

course can be attempted. It may be useful to refer readers to three accounts of knowledge and skills for community workers; each is helpful in different ways.

The Central Council for Education and Training in Social Work has published a study on 'The Teaching of Community Work'.[3] The purpose was to encourage changes in the full-time Certificate of Qualification in Social Work syllabus and so it has a heavily professional and academic bias; but its discussion of the context of community work and its explication of tasks is relevant and useful. However, it provides scope and ideas solely in the context of existing courses and institutions.

The Association of Community Workers has produced a booklet[4] which is derived from a working group of community workers and teachers It tackles only the content of training and not the means. Since it postpones questions of priority and purpose, it rather gives the impression that 'you can believe almost anything and be some sort of reasonable community worker – only find your best ideological niche'.

The Naish and Filkin pamphlet referred to earlier avoids reference to academic subject matter, disciplines, syllabus and theory, but stresses the kinds of approaches and difficulties that are likely to constrain community work whose primary activity is resource distribution. Its matter-of-fact, eyes-wide-open manner and its emphasis on organisational and group work skills make it a useful document. However, it does not get into the consideration of the theoretical and substantive knowledge needed for effective community work.

All three publications contain full inventories of the skills needed by community workers. Rather than repeat the lists or attempt an amalgamation, I will outline what I see as the important areas of knowledge for community workers. I shall then indicate that skill teaching needs to be clearly and fully related to this knowledge base. I shall argue that knowledge and skills need to be developed within the kind of direct experience model of a course outlined above, and I shall be more concerned with indicating the implications of this model than with being definitive about the knowledge and skills that are acquired within it.

KNOWLEDGE FOR COMMUNITY WORK

There are two types of knowledge useful to community workers: theoretical and substantive. Examples of theoretical knowledge are the differences between formal and operative goals in organisations, theory of the state, theory of housing classes, of reference groups, and model strategies available to community work. Examples of substantive knowledge are public health law, housing law, and the know-how needed to put out a news sheet.

There are five areas or themes where theoretical and substantive knowledge provides a context for practical skills. These involve acquiring an understanding of:

social structure and social organisations;
how organisations work;
people in their environment;
behaviour in groups;
the power structure.

1 *Understanding society*
We should help community work students to acquire what C. Wright Mills described as 'the sociological imagination'.

'The sociological imagination enables its possessor to understand the larger historical scene in terms of its meaning for the inner life and the external career of a variety of individuals. It enables him to take into account how individuals, in the welter of their daily experience, often become falsely conscious of their social positions. Within that welter the framework of modern society is sought, and within that framework the psychologies of a variety of men and women are formulated. By such means the personal uneasiness of individuals is focused upon explicit troubles and the indifference of publics is transformed into involvement with public issues.'[5]

The development of such an imagination cannot happen in a short introductory course; indeed, I would suggest that this area is so fundamental to community work for resource distribution that it needs to be seen as the spine which influences every part of a course. In my experience, it is possible for students to discuss political issues instructively; but what is also needed is a presentation of the different explanations (based on different political/ideological standpoints) of the same relevant social phenomena, relevance always being defined in terms of the students' direct experience of problems and issues. Just one example of the way in which a 'rib' can join well with this spine could be a research topic which examines some issue in depth in order to explore its ideological aspects. In this example, as with other ways of relating 'spinal content' to other parts of the course, it is necessary to avoid narrow theoretical or objective definitions; the role of the teacher should be to bring into discussion relevant conceptual schemes and to engage the students in ideological critique. The aim is to make clear to students their value assumptions, their working ideology, and how they take for granted the rightness and wrongness of alternative action possibilities.

2 *Understanding organisations*
Community workers are not likely to be able to manipulate organisations

or even protect themselves from their own employing organisations if they don't know how they work. Identifying and clarifying constraints and helping others to do the same is a continuous job, but one which has not been studied much by organisational sociologists. Many teachers do no more than parade the wares of organisational sociology (e.g. social action theory, goals, structure, communication, power).

An alternative approach is to bring out the relevance of organisation theory by helping students to examine and discuss their own experience of organisations. The use of the Brunel studies of social services departments[6] or Dorothy Smith's analysis of staff roles in psychiatric hospitals[7] can also make students far more aware of their own organisational base and of those organisations that are their targets in the resource distribution process. An organisational elucidation of local government administration is a necessary central theme for any community work course. But, whatever organisation is examined, the teacher should realise that often the best direct source of information is in the heads and experiences of the students themselves.

3 Understanding people in their environment

C. Wright Mills is again a helpful guide to this area. He helpfully distinguishes 'the personal troubles of milieu' from 'the public issues of social structure'.[8] It is the former that community work courses have conventionally tried to deal with by means of psychology or 'social psychology'. Where the adaptation of that curriculum has surely been weak is in its inability to deal effectively with the area where personal troubles become public issues, an area which is crucial to community work. Both the CCETSW and ACW booklets offer examples of this difficulty, and the latter in particular gives a full inventory of the topics which ought to be considered, and which make the individual the starting point of inquiry, moving towards the 'matters that transcend these local environments of the individual and the range of his inner life'.[9] These give support to the helpful comment from CCETSW that what is needed is 'to find the right balance between the study of psychodynamic and socio-economic theories of human behaviour'.[10]

It is interesting that, in order to suggest what is possible, the CCETSW study harks right back to Marie Jahoda's suggestion in the first Gulbenkian Report (1968) which recommended 'an eclectic approach using such key concepts as "culture (values and norms), role, status, social classes, social groups and personality" within the contexts of "changing social structures over time" '. 'Significantly,' the CCETSW notes, 'all of these terms are common to sociology and psychology.'[11] But, as a recent plea[12] to social psychologists to 'become more social' clearly shows, social psychologists have rarely studied alienation, the effects of the mass media, the experience of collective action, least of all in ways that benefit 'the down people'.

Psychologists are rarely at home in the natural settings where community workers work.

If students are to seek an understanding of the predicament and experience of working-class residents, they should study the life and consciousness of individuals, groups, and the area. How do different people feel about collective and individual action? What action has there been? How does one understand the experience of an immigrant, a single mother, a claimant, or a member of a residents' association without being one? A possible 'eclectic approach' – one which is being experimented with at Birmingham Polytechnic – is to use theories of the self (e.g. Mead, Laing, Gouldner) and consciousness (e.g. Marx, Runciman) to give an appreciation of the lives of certain individuals, groups, and settings – the young, middle-class housewives, the aged, working men and women, immigrants, life in the suburbs and the inner city – using sociological writings, first-hand written accounts, and students' experience. In this way, the traditional areas of study such as 'community', the family, subcultures, stigma, kinship, sex divisions and roles are not looked at in isolation, but in a 'real' context which should resonate in students' experiences. There is an added advantage in that a whole fertile area of study (usually called the sociology of deviance) about perceptions of groups and individuals by others may be linked in, rather than left apart like an interesting side-show.

4 Behaviour in groups
The Central Council study described three types of group situations commonly met by community workers:

'The first will involve people coming together perhaps for the first time, and with a variety of reasons for doing so, possibly for a common purpose – though this purpose may be clearer to the worker than to the group.
'The second is a group which is already formed and which may have a quite structured purpose which includes formally defined objectives, roles and responsibilities – a tenants' association committee or a local authority committee. In such a group the worker may be a stranger and he may be the person who is unclear about his role and the purpose of his presence – or he may have objectives not apparently shared by the others.
'The third is the group that is composed of representatives of other organisations. Each member will come owing prior allegiance to his own agency and may have varying degrees of ambivalence to the purposes of the group.'[13]

It follows that community workers must learn to be good at helping people to gain confidence, to tackle tasks which they wouldn't have dared tackle before, to deal with obstacles, to keep on sharpening the purpose of an informal organisation and to secure the co-operation of possible helpers. But what theoretical knowledge can help? Group theory is, in my view, treacherous ground for community work students; yet it appears to offer so much.

Group work is not a clear, coherent set of theories; but the main model implicit in most group work used in colleges is the therapeutic model used in social work. In fact, many group work tutors available to teach on college community work courses are social work staff. These tutors are not usually equipped to discuss the three types of situations described in the CCETSW report.

Some community workers have sought opportunities to understand behaviour in groups by going outside the mainstream of social group work, for instance to the encounter and sensitivity group movements. These are experimental forms of learning and would seem appropriate within the direct experience model. But many people have expressed their suspicion of training groups that claim to increase people's sensitivity. Bob Houlton, for instance, has written that:

> 'While the group sessions might be valuable to tough-minded professionals, I feel that they can be highly dangerous for activists. Too much "sensitivity" can result in timidity, nervousness and too great an awareness of personal faults. My advice would be to stay away from "T-groups", particularly if they are organised by professionals, because the result might be the increase of the powers of manipulation of the professionals, and the weakening of the activist. . . . If you want to develop your social sensitivity, it is better to do it by yourself.'[14]

Some courses have already striven to overcome this problem by starting from the students' own experience in groups of different kinds. In developing styles of action, is it not better to encourage students to write and organise simulations based on their direct experience, and for them to seek the theoretical responses and advice of a helpful group work tutor if one is available?

5 Understanding the power structure

One of the best ways to teach people about the way local government and central government work is to link it to a short research exercise of the sort described in the chapter by John Lambert, and from there to build up a political economy perspective of the home city, working out the relationships of local government to central government and the way in which the former mediates the policies of the latter. A description of the local area can get into studies of local union branches and their relationship with the national union, businesses with their parent concerns, and voluntary organisations with their central organisations. This area should not be held distinct from an area of study which is usually called social policy, and which is very difficult to teach interestingly. A social history approach (using case studies) joined with the study of formal politics, organisation studies, political theory, and a study of interventions like the Urban Programme offer opportunities to leaven social policy. Housing, education, income maintenance, race relations, employment, welfare and the health service can all be treated in this way.

It will be apparent from what has gone before that I think there is next to no community work theory *per se*, but it is important that the theoretical contributions of other disciplines should be drawn together into discussion of what should be done. One way is to discuss recorded examples of community work, like those given in the two books by David Jones and Marjorie Mayo[15] and the case studies edited by Gary Craig.[16] The theoretical work should also come home to roost in discussing the work of the students and their written accounts of what they are doing.

In exploring these foregoing areas of knowledge, I have left out examples of substantive knowledge of the sort referred to earlier. One of the main benefits of the direct experience model of training is that if the details of legislation become an important issue for students working say, on public health matters, then it *automatically* goes on the agenda. The same would apply where students needed information quickly on, for example, property law or trade union procedure in industrial disputes.

SKILLS FOR COMMUNITY WORK

In this section I propose to give examples of community work skills, indicating how they may be learned within the direct experience model. This part of the action–theory dialogue almost justifies on its own the in-action learning of a direct experience model, and it is that part which can probably be best learned by real involvement in primary community work.

Let us take two examples:

1 *The skills of Getting Information and Building up Useful Knowledge about a Task or Locality*
This relates clearly and easily to the kind of research exercise discussed by John Lambert. In this example, the theoretical input provided guidelines and background theory for a practical research exercise (conceptualising research problems, offering examples, theoretical frameworks for different approaches to fact finding) which is an important preliminary to the action exercise itself; support and de-briefing reinforces the preparation and interaction with the experience of students as they work on the problem and report back on it. In this case, the theory input and the experience of students interact and are as important as each other. The same would be true in similar examples like recording and evaluation.

2 *The Skill of Helping Groups of People to Become More Effective at Getting Tasks Done*

This needs some preparation outside the action because there is a risk that inexperienced workers may be disruptive to a group. Before they start learning in the action, they must have an opportunity to learn the bad effects of, for example, nervous assertiveness or pessimistic sympathy. But preparation is all it really is; the real learning takes place on the job. Some protagonists of full-time training make great claims for simulation, and in fact simulation, when well used, is an extremely valuable technique for reconstructing work situations which may be encountered by inexperienced would-be workers. But it can never relay all the characteristics of the real-life situation, although with the help of an organiser experienced in community work it can reproduce a surprising degree of authenticity. But used by a tutor without community work experience, with inexperienced students, it risks confirming preconceptions and acting out misleading models of action that may even unwittingly have been written into the script. It should, therefore, be regarded as a learning aid which needs to be checked out by direct experience. Subsequently, it is an important means of helping trainees to re-run experiences which they have had in action.

These examples should serve to show that, while the formal teaching situation may be able to explain or show trainees something of what the tasks are like, the real learning takes place in action. I am not here underrating the importance of many technical skills, like putting a news-sheet together, making posters, and using a duplicator or a projector; these can be taught by instruction and 'having a go'. But here, too, experience adds a crucial ingredient: when these technical skills are learnt it is what they are used for and how they are used that then becomes important.

Community work students are also expected to develop aspects of their personality useful in their work. For instance, the ACW booklet talks about the community worker's need to present him/herself as a useful person, and, while it may in some cases just add up to attempts to disguise ineffectiveness, it does point to the importance of what might be called 'style'. It is often forgotten by trainers that if a community worker cannot communicate, he's finished. But it is that skill to communicate which signifies and justifies the cumulative combination of the knowledge and theory, the skills, the clarity of objectives, the personal qualities, and the usefulness of the worker. It also indicates that not only is it important to reach a stage of being able to combine the lessons and skills learned, but also to have the ability to resolve the continual tension engendered by new information, situations, and changes of view. It is the stylistic equivalent of thinking on one's feet, which is itself an essential but difficult skill to acquire, and one which many community workers (after long years of being trained to think on paper) are quite bad at. How do you teach that in the classroom?

Students must also be helped to clarify their personal objectives. It is likely that much of the community worker's interest in training will stem from the desire to get things straight; he will ask himself such questions as: '*What* am I doing in community work? What am *I* doing in community work? What should I be doing? Where is community work going?' The personal objectives which often take a person into community work are not always those which emerge and re-emerge over several years of work. To work, as most community workers do, in a context where one's own sense of purpose is constantly buffeted by people with different life experiences and political philosophies makes it likely that the worker will either retreat into dogma or shut out criticism and soldier on regardless. Most community workers are aware that the views they hold about their purposes do affect their work and that these need constant self-criticism. But this self-criticism is exhausting and difficult, and deserves proper support. Mutual ego massage won't do. There is a role here for the teacher to become a resource person to the student/worker, that of helping the worker to make personal sense of the phenomena seen and experienced and to work over the conclusions.

CONCLUSION

In this chapter I have argued that students, if they are involved and can share a common definition of the primary tasks of community work, are the major resource for teaching material; for their experiences, values, assumptions and ideology provide that material. The course's role is to present academic concepts as possibly useful means of organising and shaping that experience so that quite self-conscious work – with justified aims, objectives, and values – can emerge.

Let us return to C. Wright Mills for a concluding comment:

'By [the use of the sociological imagination] men whose mentalities have swept only a series of limited orbits often come to feel as if suddenly awakened in a house with which they had only supposed themselves to be familiar. Correctly or incorrectly, they often come to feel that they can now provide themselves with adequate summations, cohesive assessments, comprehensive orientations. Older decisions, that once appeared sound, now seem to them products of a mind unaccountably dense. Their capacity for astonishment is made lively again. They acquire a new way of thinking, they experience a transvaluation of values: in a word, by their reflection and by their sensibility they realise the cultural meaning of the social sciences.'[17]

Without that reflection and sensibility, valuation is impossible. The purpose of training is to enable workers to know what they are doing and so to be able to evaluate it.

REFERENCES

1 Gulbenkian Foundation, *Community Work and Social Change* (Longmans, London, 1968), p. 35 (report of a study group on training).

2 Michael Naish and Elizabeth Filkin, *What does a community worker need to know? What does a community worker need to be able to do?* (University of London, Goldsmiths College, 1974), No. 2 in series 'Occasional Papers in Community & Youth Work'.

3 Central Council for Education and Training in Social Work, *Social Work Curriculum Study: The Teaching of Community Work* (London, CCETSW, 1974).

4 Association of Community Workers, *Knowledge & Skills for Community Work* (London, ACW, 1975).

5 C. Wright Mills, *The Sociological Imagination* (Harmondsworth, Pelican, 1970), p. 11.

6 Brunel University: Social Services Organisational Research Unit, *Social Service Departments: developing patterns of work and organisation* (London, Heinemann, 1974).

7 Dorothy Smith, 'Front Line Organisation of the State Mental Hospital', *Administrative Science Quarterly*, vol. 10, No. 3, December 1965, pp. 381-99.

8 C. Wright Mills, op. cit., p. 14.

9 C. Wright Mills, ibid.

10 CCETSW, op. cit., p. 34 para. 3.48.

11 CCETSW, op. cit., p. 35 para. 3.49.

12 N. Armistead (ed.), *Reconstructing Social Psychology* (Harmondsworth, Penguin Education, 1974).

13 CCETSW, op. cit., p. 44 para. 4.22.

14 Bob Houlton, *The Activist's Handbook* (London, Arrow, 1975), p. 28.

15 David Jones and Marjorie Mayo (eds), *Community Work One* and *Community Work Two* (London, Routledge & Kegan Paul, 1974 and 1975 (respectively).

16 G. Craig (ed.), *Community Work Case Studies* (Association of Community Workers, Newcastle upon Tyne, 1974).

17 C. Wright Mills, op. cit., p. 14.

PART III

DEVELOPING PRACTICE: THE STUDENT

INTRODUCTION TO PART III

There is considerable ambivalence amongst community work teachers, students and staff about the practice of placing students in a field situation in which they may take opportunities to develop their skill in, and knowledge of, community work. The ambivalence is provoked by a number of factors, including the scarcity of community workers with the experience and skills to undertake fieldwork teaching and supervision; the dangers to both students and residents of 'letting loose' students on a neighbourhood; the complexities of assessing the progress of students; and a continuing difficulty on the part of training institutions and fieldwork supervisors to delineate the areas of practice skill that they wish to see developed in their community work students.

In addition, the presence of students is a mixed blessing to the community work agency. Bill Taylor has summarised the advantages and disadvantages of taking students.* The former include:

students often bring a critical questioning of the philosophy structure and methods of work of the agency;
they are an additional source of labour;
students bring into the agency much current thinking and knowledge, as well as the results of recent research. The community work supervisor's contacts with the college, other colleagues who are also supervising and the student body may extend his horizons and deepen his knowledge and understanding.

Among the disadvantages are:

a student's approach to work may diverge from that of the agency and confuse local groups and other agencies;
students have a dual loyalty (to the agency and their college) and this may cause problems in accountability;
the supervisor may find himself involved in the internal politics of the training institution if crucial issues arise between staff and students.

The difficulties and opportunities in fieldwork placements for community work students are comprehensively discussed in the chapter by

* In a letter to the editors, 2 April 1975.

Barbara Holmes and Richard Bryant, writing from their experiences as fieldwork teachers in working class inner city areas of Glasgow. They write that '. . . the basic contribution of the fieldwork teacher . . . relates to the working relationship he can create with local leaders and organisations. The art of fieldwork teaching lies in linking this local involvement to student training in a way which benefits both the community groups and students.' Holmes and Bryant go on to discuss the aims of fieldwork placement, the practice skills to be acquired, the basic stages in the organisation and development of a placement and the role of the fieldwork teacher.

Harry Salmon discusses in detail some of the complexities in assessing students in community work placements. Warning that 'assessment is a dangerous business', he suggests that the assessment process tells us as much about the agency as the skills and competency of students. Besides describing the present situation, Salmon offers some ingredients for a model of assessment in community work placements, including the knowledge, skills and attitudes upon which students might be assessed.

One of the issues that emerges from the chapter by Salmon is the extent to which many training institutions and field supervisors rely upon methods and principles of supervision that have been developed in social casework. The interrelationships between case and community work are further explored in the chapter by Jalna Hanmer. More specifically, she examines the intrarole conflict that students experience as they move from and to placements in casework and community work. This conflict focuses on factors like the differences in the nature of their authority for intervention that students discovered in the respective roles of case and community workers, and Hanmer discusses some of the devices, such as compartmentalisation, that students use to reduce or eliminate intrarole conflict.

Chapter 10

FIELDWORK TEACHING IN COMMUNITY WORK

Barbara Holmes and Richard Bryant

The teaching of community work can be located within a variety of settings and can be organised around a range of different educational methods. Teaching settings may include the classrooms of educational establishments and fieldwork programmes which are linked with action research projects or organisations which are directly engaged in the practice of community work. Educational methods can include traditional teaching techniques, such as lectures, seminars and tutorials; innovatory methods, such as role playing and simulation games which are concerned with anticipating real life practice situations; and, finally, the use of fieldwork placements, either through the placement of students with community organisations or the organising of fieldwork assignments which are directly controlled by teaching establishments.

When we consider these settings and educational methods, it is important not to think of them as being alternatives. Each of the different teaching methods mentioned has particular strengths and weaknesses and all should, ideally, be viewed as reinforcing elements within an integrated learning process and not as options between which educationalists need to make a choice. We should also seek to avoid the stereotyped thinking which crudely assigns the teaching of practice skills exclusively to fieldwork settings and preserves classroom-centred teaching for more 'academic' pursuits. Practice-oriented teaching, particularly in the form of game and role playing, can be based within classroom situations. On the other hand, theoretical teaching and wider debates about community work – its philosophy, methods and objectives – can be organised within fieldwork situations.

In this chapter we are concerned with one of the major settings and methods for the teaching of community work – the setting provided by fieldwork agencies and the teaching of community work through the direct exposure of students to action- and practice-centred situations. The material which is presented is mainly drawn from our experience as fieldwork teachers with two community work training units which are attached to a voluntary organisation in Glasgow.[1] Both the training units are based in working-class areas in the inner city of Glasgow – the neighbouring districts of Gorbals and Govanhill – and both units attempt to perform the dual functions of student training centres and community work agencies for local organisations and residents. Since the first unit was established, in February 1971, some sixty students have completed fieldwork placements. The majority of these students have come from professional social work courses in Scotland and the main intake of students has been from the social work courses which are organised at Glasgow University. The length of fieldwork placements varies between three months on a block basis and from five to six months on a concurrent basis. The staff of the fieldwork units now comprises two fieldwork teachers, two secretaries and one community worker.

AIMS OF FIELDWORK PLACEMENTS

Social work educationalists have been frequently criticised for the vagueness which surrounds the planning, organisation and definition of fieldwork placements in community work. One particularly forceful critic, Gerry Williams, has commented:

'I think they are eager to give community work placements for the simple reason it is the "in thing", and it seemed to be something that perhaps social workers should be doing. I don't think they are altogether clear what will come out of the placement, or in what way the placement fits into the overall job that the social worker is later going to do.'[2]

We would generally agree with these criticisms and would add that similar criticisms could also be levelled against some of the community work courses and fieldwork placements which are linked with non-social work disciplines, such as youth work and adult education. It is also worth noting that, despite the recent revival of interest in community work, few educational institutions yet appear to have established a structure of staff resources, educational and community work experience and curriculum planning which is appropriate for the systematic development of community work teaching. Although there has been a rapid growth of community work teaching on British social work courses, community work still occupies a very marginal position in terms of the overall curriculum planning and resource allocation on many courses.[3]

The rather confused situation which exists on many social work courses means that fieldwork teachers and other community workers who supervise student placements can, potentially, exercise a considerable influence over the organisation and content of fieldwork training. The lack of a dominant, conventional wisdom about community work theory and the absence of any well established fieldwork traditions in community work placements can create considerable scope for innovation, and fieldworkers, as the people who are actually operating in practice-centred settings, are often better placed than many course organisers – who may not have any recent experience of 'doing' community work – to define a *modus operandi* for fieldwork training. In the Glasgow units, the fieldwork teachers have the primary responsibility for not only supervising the student's work in the placement situation, but also for deciding what varieties and styles of community work the student will experience. The degree of influence and direction exercised by many training establishments over the fieldwork process can be very limited. This situation reflects, in part, the lack of definition of course objectives in relation to community work placements and, in more practical terms, the absence of any ongoing and sustained contacts between the educational establishments and fieldwork agencies. Whether the fieldworker's mode of operation and style of community work practice fits with the assumptions of course organisers and students is sometimes a rather hit-and-miss affair.[4]

We would suggest that two related objectives are appropriate for community work placements.

1 The use of community work placements to provide social work students with a basic introduction to how particular community work agencies operate and the types and range of issues, problems and controversies which can influence the activities of full-time workers and local residents. Here the educational emphasis is not on the direct acquisition of practice skills. The emphasis is on the student gaining some general insights into the mechanics and functions of community work, insights which (one hopes) may be of some value in the student's future work in a variety of social work settings. This may include, for instance, developing ideas about how local authority social workers might link up more effectively with self-help groups and gaining practical insights into just how long-term and time-consuming is the community work commitment which is needed for the development of some local initiatives. Also, the problem on which local community organisations are active can, at times, provide students with first-hand insights into wider political and social policy issues. For instance, students with the Glasgow units are invariably in contact, at some stage of their placement, with the complex and often bitter political debates about housing in the city.

Observational placements which provide students with an overview of an agency and some of its activities can be particularly useful for students – like many who come to the Glasgow units – who have had little or no previous experiences of working with community groups and community work agencies. Whether this observational activity is, at some stage in the placement, linked with more practice-centred tasks depends mainly upon the length of the student's placements.

2 The use of fieldwork placements for the teaching of practice skills in

community work. The move from observational learning – which is mainly geared to providing insights into the work of particular agencies – into the direct teaching of practice skills takes us into a more problematic and potentially more controversial area of fieldwork training. When we talk about practice skills in community work, we are essentially concerned with the basic ingredients of 'doing' community work: the arts, techniques, information and insights community workers need and how they organise and apply their knowledge and experience in action situations. How educationalists conceptualise and define practice skills will be influenced by a variety of factors, such as the value assumptions they hold about the nature and function of community work, the work experiences they had in different organisational and social settings and the perspectives they have on the relationship between community work and other forms of planned interventions (including social case-work).

It is over questions like the defining of practice skills in community work that the vagueness and confusion about community work which exists on many social work courses becomes very apparent. We have rarely received from course organisers a well defined set of guidelines for the teaching of practice skills which are geared specifically to com-munity work placements, rather than being based on models derived from casework or youth work experiences. While some of the experiences and skills which are considered as important in social casework are certainly relevant to community work placements – particularly in the development of interpersonal relationships – it is very questionable whether conventional models of casework skills can be projected, in a wholesale fashion, into the arena of community work education. One obvious gap, which a number of community workers have commented upon, is the lack of emphasis which is given in some models of casework skills to organisational, social planning and political activities. Because of our dissatisfaction with models which conceptualise community work as casework multiplied by x, we have – like some other fieldwork teachers – attempted to identify a range of skills which are more appropriate and relevant to community work activities. These skills are defined under six related headings:[5]

(a) *Engagement skills:* e.g. establishing working relations with staff, local residents and community leaders, being able to function in unstructured and sometimes chaotic situations, use of self and self-awareness in action situations;

(b) *Organisational skills:* e.g. developing a grasp of the mechanics and dilemmas of building organisations, work with committees and organising public events;

(c) *Planning and policy skills:* e.g. analysis of issues and problems, ability to generalise from the specific, relating individual grievances to organisational responses, evaluation of work completed;

(d) *Action skills:* e.g. ability to work towards specific objectives, ability to make decisions in situations where all the relevant information is never available, 'plotting out' strategic and tactical options and their possible implications for action initiatives;

(e) *Communication skills:* e.g. communicating with others by written and spoken word, ability to adjust style and manner of communication according to different situational contexts:

(f) *Political skills:* e.g. ability to view local initiatives within a broader socio-economic framework of reference, a knowledge of the sociology of political decision making and a grasp of different varieties of political ideologies and their implications for change-centred action, ability to work within a political framework.

These skills can obviously be used and applied in a variety of community work settings. A key question arises over the emphasis and weighting which is given to the possible range and combinations of tasks which can be included under any of these headings. For instance, under 'engagement' and 'organisational' skills, we would not emphasise – in contrast to many community work educationalists – the ability to perform mediator and broker tasks between community groups and local or central government departments. This is because we feel that community workers are basically in business to encourage the development of organisations which will directly express the interests of their members and should not act as a link between formal organisations and their 'publics'. Even in a simple typology, like the one we have outlined, the range of skills mentioned is idealised. No student or community worker is ever likely to be of equal competence and ability in all these skills. Thus, when we come to passing judgment on students – as, for instance, in the final evaluation and assessment of a fieldwork placement – we are almost inevitably going to have, in the back of our minds, some sort of ranking order of practice skills. Because we have a bias towards a community action approach to community work, our own personal ranking order tends to place a priority on the development of organising skills and, in the words of C. W. Mills, the ability to relate 'private troubles to public ills'.

THE ORGANISATION OF PLACEMENTS: BASIC STAGES

Community work placements, like local community work initiatives, rarely develop in a spontaneous manner. The orientation, style and content of a placement is invariably conditioned by an often complex decision-making process which may involve a wide number of individuals and organisations. The principal participants are likely to include the field-worker and his or her employing agency, the course organisers, the student and local activists and their organisations. As was previously noted, in our experience the fieldwork teacher often plays the dominant role in this decision-making process and his or her influence is normally felt throughout the history of a placement. We would distinguish four basic stages in the organisation and history of a placement,[6] which can often overlap and become rather blurred in the fieldwork situation.

1 Pre-placement Planning

Of particular importance during the pre-placement stage is the contact which is established between the fieldwork agency and educational estab-lishments and the planning which is undertaken in the local situation by the fieldwork teacher. The contact between the fieldwork agency and the educational establishment should include, at a minimum, joint preparatory meetings between the fieldwork teacher, the student and the course organiser to consider the student's previous work experience, the course organiser's expectations about the placement and a general review of the activities with which the fieldwork agency is currently involved, and an outline of the possible types of work the student might be engaged in. This basic preparation has been a regular feature of our contact with the courses at Glasgow University, but has often been lacking with place-ments which are linked with other universities and colleges. One simple factor, which has limited joint planning exercises with a number of educa-tional establishments which are not based in Glasgow, has been the physical distance which separates some educational establishments from the local fieldwork situation. Distance and the limited time available for travelling have, in some cases, severely restricted the opportunity for tutors, fieldworkers and students to get together both prior to the start of a placement and during the actual period of a placement.

With the Glasgow units, the pre-placement planning in the local situation normally involves the fieldwork teacher – sometimes, but not always, in consultation with local activists – deciding upon the main area of work the student will tackle and designing a tentative outline for the organisation of a placement. At this stage, our local planning rarely involves the working-out of a detailed agenda for the placement; rather it involves making general decisions about what groups or issues the students will be involved with. During the early placements with our first fieldwork unit, we asked the students themselves to choose between a number of potential placement alternatives, such as work with local tenants' groups, assisting with the organisation of the community news-paper for the Gorbals and Govanhill area or exploring felt needs and leadership resources in a particular neighbourhood. But experience has indicated that this is a rather unrealistic policy, since few students when they are preparing for a placement have either the knowledge or the background experience to make a clear-cut selection. Now the fieldwork teacher initially defines and specifies an area of work for the student, on the understanding that this decision may be reviewed and revised if the early stages of the placement reveal any major difficulties about a particular assignment.

2 Student Orientation

Although the students who come to the Glasgow units commence their placements within a structured framework, they are not expected to move straight into action- and practice-centred situations. Students have tended to find the first weeks of their placement with the Glasgow units difficult as they attempt to define and discover roles for themselves, adjust to the ethos and organisation of the fieldwork units and assimilate information about the agency, local areas and the activities and histories of the community groups with whom they will be working. The first stage of the placement is very much an orientation period for the student and during this time a considerable emphasis is placed upon observational work and learning. This period is also generally one of the most time-consuming for the fieldwork teacher, as the fieldwork teacher must often be available for consultation to a much greater extent than is the case later on in a placement. Where there is a group of students already on placement, the initial orientation stage may become less stressful for the new student, because a considerable amount of background information and support can be provided by the other students. The ideal situation has been one where placements have been staggered and overlap occurs. For instance, work on a continuing project is passed on from one student to another and the students concerned normally have a strong commitment to pass on and receive relevant background material and generally to help facilitate a smooth introduction for the new student.

3 Task-centred Activity

If a fieldwork placement is intended to provide a student with some degree of practice experience in community work, then a decision has to be made, at some stage, about the specific nature of the tasks and activities the student will be involved in. The transition from the observation to the task-centred stage normally occurs, with the Glasgow units, after the first month of a placement, although in some exceptional circumstances the students have moved into direct practice roles at a much earlier stage of their placement.[7] This shift into the task-centred stage of a placement – where the emphasis is placed on working directly with local groups on particular action initiatives – involves the student in a narrowing of their work focus and demands that a more detailed and coherent programme of work is devised by the fieldwork teacher and the student. For instance, a student who has been, during his initiation period, working generally with a local tenants' group – attending meetings, talking to key activists, familiarising himself with the group's past activities – may narrow his work to focus on one particular issue or problem with which the local organisations are concerned, e.g. complaints about dampness in council flats, a local fund-raising campaign, attempts to recruit new members in a newly built part of an estate. Wherever possible, decisions about the selection of particular tasks or projects are taken in consultation with the local community groups and leaders.[8]

4 Student Withdrawal and Evaluation

The final stage of the placement – the withdrawal of the student from the local situation and the final evaluation and assessment of a placement – requires very careful planning. One of the basic dilemmas in many community work placements involves the risk that a student will build up local work commitments which are left 'up in the air' at the end of the placement or that new projects will be started which may collapse once a placement finishes. Pre-placement planning can help to minimise these risks, although no fieldwork teacher is ever likely to be in a position to predict and budget for all the practical outcomes and possible action implications of student placements. Attempting to ensure that a continuity of local work is maintained between student placements and that commitments made in a placement are not lost or neglected has been one of the major concerns with the Glasgow fieldwork units. The employment of a full-time community worker, in August 1973, helped considerably in ensuring continuity but it is still necessary for the fieldwork teacher to keep in close touch with the local work of students. They need to have local links, to be able to pick up on developments and provide a stable reference and contact point for the local leaders. As with the initial orientation stage, having a group of students together on placements and having an overlap between placements can also be a considerable advantage during the final period of a placement.

Overlap between placements facilitates the handing over of contacts, information and commitments from one student to another and also helps the fieldwork agency to sustain a continuity in the services and support provided to local groups. With the Glasgow units, this linking-up between placements has also been helped by the fact that the fieldwork units have been mainly engaged in working on a small number of comparatively long-term local involvements rather than a larger number of one-off initiatives. For example, the units' work with a tenants' association in one of the redevelopment areas in Govanhill has covered a two-year period, during which time the tenants' association has had an involvement with a total of eight different student placements. This long-term contact has enabled the fieldwork teacher with our Govanhill unit, the community worker, and the leaders of the tenants' association to work out a detailed *modus operandi* on the role and function of students with this association.

It should also be noted that the preparation of the final evaluation and assessment for a placement can also require a considerable time and planning commitment for the fieldwork teacher and the student. The policy in the Glasgow units is to commence preparing for the final evaluation two or three weeks before the end of a placement and to work towards the completion of any written material and reports during the final week of a placement.

We would not wish to claim that these four stages provide universal guidelines for the organisation of community work placement or that the same stages are necessarily relevant to all types of community work placement. What we would suggest, on the basis of our experience, is that community work placements do need to be carefully organised and that a structured approach is more desirable than a *laissez-faire* or 'do-it-yourself' approach which places students in agencies and local areas with the minimum of back-up support, guidance and planning.

LEARNING SITUATIONS AND TEACHING METHODS

Throughout all the stages of a placement, opportunities should arise for the student to gain some insight into the practice of community work and, especially during the activity-centred stage of a placement, some experience of directly working with local community groups. When we consider the various learning situations which can be generated during a placement and the various teaching methods which can be used, it is useful to distinguish between those learning situations and teaching methods which can be directly initiated and set up by the fieldwork teacher and those learning situations which can emerge more informally and spontaneously as a result of the student's interaction with local groups, community leaders and other activists in practice situations. In the Glasgow units we attempt to provide students with a basic structure of formally organised learning situations, which are primarily concerned with examining either the student's work with local groups or wider issues which arise from the ongoing activities of the fieldwork units. These include:

Supervision Sessions
These meetings between a fieldwork teacher and individual students are held on either a weekly or a fortnightly basis. While variations naturally occur according to the people involved, there is a marked tendency for these supervisory sessions to concentrate mainly on the activities of local groups and the student's role in relation to them rather than upon the

student's own personal motivations and characteristics. Gerry Williams has commented that, in his experience of student supervision in community work, there is a strong emphasis on 'practical work'[9] and this is certainly reflected in the supervision sessions which are held in the Glasgow units. The focal points for discussion in these supervisory sessions are often provided by material which is drawn from the recordings which are made by students during their placements. Students are asked to keep a brief daily log of their activities and to review, at the end of each month, the use of their time, their most difficult experiences and their goals for the coming month. They are also required to keep a report of every local meeting they attend, which covers such points as the group's business, the main speakers and the student's own role in the meetings. Some students have found this style of recording poses problems for them, as they have never previously been accountable in such detail for the use of their time nor have had to establish clearly their priorities between competing issues and demands. Students also record their personal goals for the placement, write their own self-evaluation and produce an evaluation of the agency.

Group Discussions
These sessions, which involve all the students who are on placement and the community work staff of the units, developed out of the weekly staff meetings for the units. Students have found these staff meetings[10] informative but felt that insufficient opportunity existed for issues to be examined in depth and for students to compare their placement experiences. When the two fieldwork units have their full intake of students, there can be as many as eight students on placement at any one time and they can be working with five or six different projects and community organisations in the Gorbals and Govanhill areas. Group discussions are now held at fortnightly intervals and, as with the individual supervision session, the emphasis is mainly placed on examining current activities and wider issues which arise from the students' involvement with local groups. Some recent topics for group discussion have included: 'Who benefits from student placements?', 'What lessons can be learned for community work theory from the Laurieston and Govanhill units?', 'Politics and community work' and 'Local associations as representatives of the community'.

Informal Contact
In terms of the overall contact between the fieldwork teachers and the students, these formally organised group and supervisory sessions only represent one type of communication during a placement. As the Glasgow fieldwork units are small organisations with a relatively non-bureaucratic style of operating, fieldwork teacher – student contact occurs throughout most days of a placement and much of the actual business of organising a placement – passing on information, arranging meetings, discussing

tactics for future activities – occurs informally because the fieldwork teacher and the student are working together in the same office and often attend the same local meetings and events in the evenings.

Outside Learning Situations
When we move outside of the environment of the fieldwork agency, we enter into a far more unstructured and unpredictable training setting. Within the agency, the fieldwork teacher can, to a considerable degree, direct and manage learning situations whereas in the wider context of working with local groups the fieldwork teacher's influence over the process and content of events is strictly limited. It would be rather alarming if this was not the case. If a fieldwork teacher could, to a considerable degree, control local events – attempting to structure the organisation of action initiatives according to educational requirements – this would mean that the fieldwork teacher and his agency were exercising the dominant influence within a locality, something which would be contrary to all the basic principles and articles of faith of community work.

It is important to stress the unpredictability which can characterise learning situations during the activity-centred stage of placement. A student might be assigned to a particular project or community group in the expectation that they might contribute to a particular local development and be exposed to certain types of learning situations and then events occur in the local situation which radically change the direction of the placement. This point can be illustrated by the experiences of a student who was assigned to work with a newly formed group in the Oatlands district of Gorbals. It was anticipated that the student would be heavily involved in providing back-up support and encouragement for the group, but events which occurred in the internal organisation of the group precipitated a crisis which required the student to play a far more activist and leadership role. The following is an extract from the student's fieldwork report:

'Because of the age of the Oatlands Community Group (less than six months), it required a lot of support and it had been one of the unit's main tasks to provide this. Between the last student who had worked with the group leaving and my taking over, there elapsed a period of four weeks during which the group had no external support and during this time it began to disintegrate. The other main factor contributing to this disintegration was the nature of the group itself, which included a married couple and the mother-in-law, on a committee of five main movers. It was here that I came on the scene and began to try to re-activate enthusiasm and reconvene the group. This seemed to have some success initially and plans were going ahead with the organisation of a public meeting to discuss the Treatment Area plans under the 1969

Housing (Scotland) Act. The relevant officials had been invited, together with the architect and local councillors. The local church agreed to the use of the hall. Four or five days prior to the meeting I was informed that the Committee had decided to resign en masse. The chairman refused to chair the meeting and having previously promised to help arrange distribution of the leaflets, opted out of this as well. Having thought for a moment of calling the whole thing off, I distributed most of the leaflets myself and enlisted a local shopkeeper to chair the meeting on a "one-off" basis. Despite this sudden crisis the meeting was very well attended, by more than 400 people, who asked many questions which suggested that some form of residents' association might still be useful. To prepare for this, I handed each person who attended a duplicated sheet explaining what the meeting was about and asking for names to form a committee. I was a little disappointed that only a dozen or so left their names. However, I decided that these might be enough to get something off the ground and convened a meeting of these people on the Sunday following the public meeting.'[11]

The Oatlands Committee resigned just before a public meeting at which all local councillors and the official in charge of the area had agreed to speak. For officialdom in Glasgow to attend such a meeting, on a Sunday, in a local area, was in itself a breakthrough. The fieldwork teacher's work in the area during the previous six months had demonstrated to her that local people were very concerned about the future of the area and a previous meeting called by the Corporation had been attended by more than 500 people. The fieldwork teacher therefore felt that the action required from her should not be to cancel the meeting but should be to ensure that local people knew of the meeting and that a local leader should chair the meeting. The student, on her direction, ensured that the necessary contacts were made. Whether or not the student unit continued to be involved in Oatlands was totally dependent on the meeting: if there was a poor turn-out the project would be dropped unless local people in the future requested help. The excellent turn-out at the meeting confirmed our impression that there was concern in the area but that as yet there was no organisation whereby this concern could be expressed. Since these developments, with support from the student unit, a viable residents' association has emerged in the area.

The example of the Oatlands group clearly illustrates the changes which can occur in local situations and how these changes may affect the student's involvement with a group and the type of learning experience he might gain. However, it should be stressed that the unpredictability of a placement experience and the changes which can occur in the student's role can vary according to the situational context in which a student is functioning. The following factors seem to be particularly influential in determining the element of unpredictability in a placement and in shaping the type of learning situations which may occur.

1 The Newness of the Local Group

Community groups which are at an early stage in their organisational development are – like all forms of organisation – more prone to shifts and changes in their leadership, policies and style of working. A student with a new organisational initiative is, invariably, in a more fluid and open placement situation than is a student who is working with an established group which has developed certain modes and habits of operating. In our experience, the outcome of a placement which is focused on new initiatives – like the Oatlands example – is usually difficult to predict. What can be noted is that placements with newly established groups often offer the student more direct experiences of local organising, especially in terms of contact work with local residents, setting up public meetings and working with emerging local leadership.

2 The Experience of Local Leadership

Community groups vary in their leadership, particularly with regard to the degree of previous organisational and leadership experience of their active members. Some of the community groups we are working with have very experienced leaders, with a background of activism in trade unions, the Labour Party, the Communist Party or voluntary groups associated with particular churches. Other groups have a leadership which is entirely composed of people who are new to organisational involvements and who have never previously sat on committees, organised public meetings, lobbied councillors or planned collective activities. While it would be misleading to suggest that experienced leaders do not need support and encouragement, it is often the case that a new leadership may require considerable back-up assistance and may be more prone to a collective loss of confidence, organisational set-backs and individual tensions as people begin to realise some of the implications (e.g. for their domestic routines) of being regularly involved in events and meetings. Students working with a group which has an inexperienced leadership are often in more volatile and unpredictable placement situations than are students whose main contact is with an experienced local leadership.

3 The Issues and Problems which concern Local Groups

The issues and problems which provide the focal points for local action can determine the way in which a group operates in terms of its strategies and policies, the timetable for action and the interactions which occur between the local group and other organisations. A number of the housing groups in the redevelopment areas of Govanhill and Gorbals operate in crisis situations and are involved in a more or less constant lobbying of councillors, local government officials and other bodies which have a responsibility for their areas. Organising in a situation where the social and physical fabric of an area is falling apart at the seams obviously creates certain pressures and demands which are largely absent from those areas – such as the new housing estates in the Hutchesontown district of Gorbals – which have a more settled population and where the residents (despite many other problems) are not confronted with living in dangerous buildings, bargaining for rehousing and the gradual disintegration of the local social system. In our experience, students who work with groups in redevelopment areas are often exposed to a more unpredictable set of circumstances – largely due to the crisis focus of work in these areas – than are students who work with some of the tenants associations on the new corporation housing estates. They also tend to be more involved, during their placement, with the politics of housing in Glasgow and conflict situations which involve the local authority.

Because of these and other factors, the learning situations which are generated during the activity-centred stage of a placement are more unstructured and unpredictable than those which can be set up within the context of the fieldwork agency. Much depends on the prevailing circumstances, the student's own use of situations and the fieldworker's contact with the ongoing process of events and his knowledge of the work of local organisations.

Although it is difficult to predict the activist functions a student might perform on a placement, it should be noted that during the activity-centred stage of a placement – even if the student is relatively passive in action terms – considerable scope should always exist for learning through observation. Observational learning on community work placements can occur at two levels: the gaining of general insights into how an agency operates (cf. above) and the direct observation of particular practice situations. Community work, unlike much of social casework, offers many and varied opportunities for students to learn through the direct observation of events and action situations. Much of community work, particularly at the neighbourhood level, does take place in public situations and many of the issues on which community workers are active are concerned with 'non-confidential' areas of activity, such as housing problems, lack of recreational amenities and planning programmes. These are discussed and acted upon in settings which are frequently open to the outside observer, such as public meetings, committee meetings and organised events in local areas. Apart from the observation of public events and meetings, the activity-centred stage of a placement should also provide opportunities for students to observe, at first hand, full-time workers and local activists operating in various action situations. In community work placements, the fieldwork teacher and student are, in our experience, frequently involved as joint participants in the same action situations and this affords obvious opportunities for both direct learning experience and follow-up teaching which focus on the 'how' and 'why' of particular developments.

THE ROLE OF THE FIELDWORK TEACHER

Throughout this article we have made repeated reference to the position and role of the fieldwork teacher. We would like to conclude by summarising the three major roles which the fieldworkers perform with the Glasgow fieldwork units.

1 Supervising Students during their Placements with the Units
This involves such activities as planning the initial programme of the placement, introducing the student to the locality and the agency, organising individual and group discussions, being available for more informal day-to-day consultation and the final assessment and evaluation of the student's placement.

2 Contact and Links with Educational Establishments
The fieldwork teacher is invariably a key factor in the linking of fieldwork placement and educational establishments and, because of this, in any effort to integrate the theoretical and practice dimensions in community work education. Activities in this linking-up process may involve attempts to establish regular meetings with course tutors which focus, in particular, upon course content and fieldwork expectations; the fieldwork teacher contributing to the teaching on courses and regular feedback to educational establishments about developments in the fieldwork situation.

3 Engaging in Community Work with Local Organisations and Projects
In the local situation the fieldwork teacher occupies the dual role of student supervisor and community worker and is constantly faced with the tensions and potential contradictions which are inherent in this position. How one attempts to reconcile the roles of neighbourhood worker/activist and fieldwork supervisor/educator presents the most demanding and crucial test for the fieldwork teacher. The role of the fieldwork teacher requires a different set of priorities in the use of time and this means that the fieldwork teacher cannot often devote all his energies to a single local issue which requires sustained personal commitment, e.g. helping to represent tenants at a valuation appeal which may drag on for several months. This tension in roles becomes crucial when we consider credibility in the area. The community workers with the Glasgow units have no statutory power and are dependent on acceptance by people in the local area in order to be able to work. Initial acceptance is greatly facilitated by being able to offer technical assistance, such as duplicating facilities, but in order to

maintain this credibility the worker must maintain links with key leaders in the area. This takes time, but it is mandatory. Although the student's acceptance or rejection by a local group ultimately depends on his own merits, his initial acceptance depends on the acceptance of the fieldwork teacher and the student unit. The continuing contact is also necessary in order to perform a 'bridging' community work role to provide some form of continuity between placements.

We feel that the tension for the fieldwork teacher of the neighbourhood activist/educator roles is healthy, but must be kept at a reasonable level. Similarly, the tension for the student of the activist/learner roles must be kept within certain limits. For this to be possible, it is essential that there is back-up support provided by full-time community work staff in addition to the support provided by the fieldwork teacher. We should not, however, seek to remove these tensions completely, as they help to prevent student units from becoming rather precious educational settings which are detached from the conflicts and confusions which so often occur in the practice of community work.

In all these roles and activities the basic contribution of the fieldwork teacher – the contribution which provides the foundation on which other developments are dependent – relates to the working relationship he can create with local leaders and organisations. The art of fieldwork teaching lies in linking this local involvement to student training in a way which benefits both the community groups and students.

NOTES AND REFERENCES

1 For a description of the early work of the first fieldwork unit which was established see B. Holmes, R. Bryant and D. Houston, 'Student Unit in Community Work: An Experimental Approach', *Social Work Today*, vol. 4, No. 10 (1973).

2 G. Williams, 'Supervision in Community Work Placements', *Aberdeen Association of Social Service*, p. 18 (1972).

3 For evidence of this see *Current Issues in Community Work* (London, Routledge & Kegan Paul, 1973).

4 See R. Bryant, 'Fieldwork Training in Community Work', *Community Development Journal*, vol. 9, No. 3 (1974).

5 We would not claim any originality for this typology of skills. It is based upon a model suggested by Prof. Slavin. See J. Rothman and W. Jones, *A New Look at Field Instruction* (New York, Association Press, 1971), p. 69.

6 We are referring here to the organisation of those placements which are sufficiently long to provide the opportunity for students to engage in some direct work with local groups.

7 This has sometimes occurred when a student has had previous community work experience and has had the knowledge and confidence to move quickly into local work situations.

8 One of the major criticisms we would level against our own work is that we have not, to date, formally involved local residents in the management of student placements. Local involvement is still at the informal level of discussion and consultation.

9 G. Williams, op. cit.

10 These staff meetings are attended by all members of the unit, including secretarial staff, and the roles of chairman and minutes secretary are rotated on a weekly basis.

11 J. Cameron, 'Placement Report' (1972).

Chapter 11

EVALUATING AND ASSESSING COMMUNITY WORK STUDENTS

Harry Salmon

Assessment is a dangerous business. It is fraught with difficulties, many of which cannot be removed from the process. There is a good deal of criticism by those being assessed of the way in which the exercise is carried out and of the criteria which are used.

In social work considerable stress is placed on assessment. A candidate is assessed as to his or her suitability for social work. The applicant for a place on a course is assessed to determine whether he or she is the *right kind* of person to benefit from that particular course. And, having gained a place on a social work qualifying course, the student is then subjected to a procedure which includes an assessment on each fieldwork placement. Often a fieldwork assessment says almost as much about the assessor as about the student. It betrays the strengths, values, prejudices and interests of the supervisor in the same language that is used to describe the performance of the student in the field. 'The student was able to link the client's behaviour with early childhood and parental attitudes' implies that the supervisor had a commitment to a particular diagnostic model just as 'The student built up a comprehensive picture of the situation which took into account social and political factors' indicates that the supervisor had a leaning towards a structural analysis of society.

In the same way, comments in an assessment can say more about the style and policy of the agency than about the student. Many of these comments are ambiguous. 'Miss X did not become integrated into the staff' might say something about Miss X or it could be saying something about the relationships within the office. A statement like 'The student found it hard to be open about his feelings in supervision sessions' might say something about the intrapersonal dynamics of the student but equally it might be an unconscious comment on the ethos of the agency or the personality of the supervisor. Again the absence of any reference to a student's ability or lack of ability to draw connections between the problems of individuals and the structural problems of society could imply either that the student was unaware of the need to establish connections or that the style of the agency was such that problems were interpreted within a policy of providing help and therapy for individuals or families.

A cynical interpretation of assessment could be that it is a game we play. Student, course tutor, supervisor and sometimes the client or community group collude at keeping within the tacitly accepted rules of the game. There must be some positive comments under particularly sensitive headings but without one or two mildly critical remarks – 'Miss S has a slight reluctance to write formal reports' – the assessment would be unreal. Here and there we must give indications of progress during the placement and if an identified weakness from a previous placement can be picked up, then that is a prize: 'During the placement, Y has overcome his former diffidence and has shown increasing confidence in his relationships with colleagues.'

Some clients or community groups begin to discern the 'rules' and are supportive of the worker. They do not make life too difficult for the student and often make approving comments to those they perceive as being responsible for the student's work.

The course tutor begins to sense when an assessment is likely to contain statements which will not fall within the rules of the game. (Experience suggests that danger signals are emitted by suggestions of 'identification with clients' or 'non-coping tendencies'.) Attempts are made – hopefully involving the student – to see whether the final assessment can be worded in such a way as to avoid putting the student's future in jeopardy. In all but a minority of instances a formula is arrived at which satisfies the external assessor. Another problem is associated with who makes up the rules. Some would argue that students can be the victims of 'supervisors' eccentricities'.[1] Certainly students are in a vulnerable position and – at the most – have a marginal influence upon the criteria of assessment and on the way the game is played.

SOME PROBLEMS IN ASSESSMENT

The whole process could be described in a more positive way but there is sufficient ground for unease to justify a de-bunking exercise. Some of the mystique which surrounds assessment needs to be dispelled – especially when you remember all the chance factors associated with placements (e.g. choice of agency, the situation within the agency, supervisors and changes in supervision arrangements, work opportunities, cases terminating unexpectedly, groups ceasing to function or external events preventing further useful intervention). In America and in this country considerable stress has been placed on field experience as a preparation for the practice of community work.[2] One of the problems, however, in both countries has been to provide enough suitable placements which also have adequate supervision. The American response to this problem has been to move in the direction of linking field instruction more directly with the teaching institutions. They are doing this in several ways – by faculties employing their own supervisors, by running field laboratory units, by schools of social work setting up their own training centres and by students being attached to agencies but supervised by university staff.[3]

It might be that we will have to experiment along similar lines, though the study group set up by the Central Council for Education and Training in Social Work had reservations about any move in this direction.[4]

At the moment, standards of supervision in community work vary tremendously[5] and consequently this creates anomalies in the assessment of students. Supervisors come from a variety of backgrounds, have differing attitudes towards assessment and hold diverse views about the relationship of community work to social work.[6] These differences introduce further elements of chance into the assessments that are likely to be made on students. The implications are even more serious if the teaching institution insists on a form of grading or the allocating of marks.

A problem of another kind is the way in which the knowledge that an assessment has to be done at the end of the placement creates an anxiety in most students to produce 'results'.[7] Often neither the work situation nor the length of the placement allow natural developments to take place. No matter how much reassurance is given, the feeling lingers in the minds of most students that they must have something to show for their intervention – a new group, an expanded committee, more involvement of local people, a successful playscheme or public meeting. The danger is that the anxiety leads to directive and manipulative behaviour which it is not always easy to bring to light in supervision sessions.

It is apparent that attitudes towards assessment vary and that these variations must affect the assessment process. Supervisors, students and course tutors can collude in such a way that the activity can generate an aura and sense of occasion. On the other hand, the same kind of collusion can take place to devalue the whole process and reduce it to something which has got to be engaged in so as to satisfy external bodies. Neither of these extremes is desirable but the position is even worse if the parties to the assessment process hold widely differing attitudes towards it. Broad agreement about the purpose and degree of importance attached to the exercise is a prerequisite for the completion of the assessment.

COURSE EXPECTATIONS

An important element in the relationship between the teaching institution and the agency is that of interpreting the expectations of the former to the latter and the transmitting of information about the opportunities and constraints within the agency. It is no use, for instance, the course sending students believing that the agency can provide a broad range of experience if, in fact, most of its current work is in one limited sphere. Or again, it is no use students arriving at the agency believing that they will have a choice of projects if this is not the case. The expectations of the course must be related to the real situation in the field.

Course expectations are often expressed in their fieldwork handbooks and categories of assessment. The extent to which these can be met vary will from place to place and will be determined by how far the assessment headings are matched to the style and policy of the agency. A fieldwork supervisor in community work often has a different approach to his task from that of a casework supervisor and finds it hard to carry out an assessment under categories which were originally devised for assessing students in casework agencies.[8]

There are wide variations between social work courses in the amount of guidance and information given to fieldwork supervisors and also in the demands they make in respect of assessment. Some courses bury supervisors under a great weight of papers while others send out the flimsiest of details. Others provide very detailed headings under which the evaluation of the students should be carried out and – for good measure – supplement these with squared charts which also should be filled in. A few leave it to the supervisor to present the assessment in his own way.

Most students are still coming into community work placements from courses which are geared primarily to casework. This means that the placement is seen as an introduction to community work rather than as a preparation for the practice of it. After all, seconding agencies are expecting to receive back caseworkers rather than community workers! All this adds to the difficulties of assessment.[9]

An article in *Case Con*,[10] to which we have already referred, strongly criticises fieldwork supervision and challenges the assumptions behind some of the evaluation guidelines. Though what is said does not always apply, and applies less than it used to, it is true that casework-oriented courses often use concepts and make assumptions which are sometimes not acceptable to a community worker.

It is, for instance, frequently implied that the worker should have co-operative relationships both within and outside the agency, that he should have a professional identity and be prepared to conform to laid down procedures. The community worker may not think the last two very important and would say of the first that it depends upon the circumstances. The student is sometimes encouraged to look critically at his agency, but he is not expected to challenge its policy. Criticism must be within the basic assumption that what the agency is doing is right. There may be scope for minor improvements in the delivery of services or adjustments in the allocation of resources but the general policy must be accepted. The community worker, however, may feel that he should criticise basic policy decisions or work with groups whose aims are to change the agency in some way.

Evaluation guidelines produced by courses which continue to be concerned mainly with casework do not, generally speaking, make provision for assessing students' political, organisational, and strategy-formulation skills.

AREAS OF PERFORMANCE

In writing about evaluation, Priscilla Young[11] identifies three areas of performance which need to be assessed. These are to do with skills, attitudes and the application of theoretical knowledge. She also goes on to emphasise that the assessment is of the student's fieldwork and not of the student as a person. Personal characteristics are only relevant when they prevent the worker functioning effectively. This is a welcome comment for it is not unusual for psycho-analytically oriented supervisors to probe into the student's relationships with his parents or siblings without a good reason. Uncomplicated students have frequently commented – sometimes light-heartedly but often with distaste – on the type of approach by a previous supervisor. In community work, personal traits tend only to be discussed when they detract seriously from a student's capacity to operate adequately. If for instance, a student is so shy and withdrawn that he cannot function in a group situation, then this has to be discussed.

The areas of performance – skills, attitudes and knowledge – offer a framework equally for assessing casework, group work or community work. What is included, however, under each heading will vary considerably according to which is the primary method of intervention being used. This is probably the point at which we should comment on evaluation guidelines provided by courses specialising in community work.

The first thing is to recognise that, though we often criticise the evaluation guidelines produced for casework placements, we have not so far established clear criteria for the assessment of students practising community work. Though the number of courses specialising in community work is still comparatively small, the range of procedures and formats for assessment is wide. At least one course has not yet felt able to set down any criteria. Another places the emphasis on self-assessment. Some offer four or five fairly general headings under which supervisors are invited to comment and others provide lengthy checklists. In view of all the uncertainty which still exists about the scope of community work practice and therefore what constitutes the appropriate body of knowledge and necessary skills, it is not surprising that there is a lack of clarity when it comes to defining categories of assessment.

A large number of skills are identified ranging from keeping accounts to ability to work in a political framework. With some thought, the skills enumerated in evaluation guidelines could be reduced to several broad headings.

The area of attitudes is the most difficult one. This is partly because it is closely related to skills but mainly because it moves into the subjective realm where assessment is particularly hazardous and controversial. This becomes particularly clear if we quote two specific references to attitudes from different evaluation outlines. One asks for a comment on student's attitude towards authority and the other for a comment on 'attitude towards assignment'. Both are value-laden. So are references like 'acceptability as a professional worker' which often figure in casework evaluation headings.

References to the application of theoretical knowledge are usually included but as a general heading. 'Ability to relate theory to practice' is the favourite phrase. The areas of knowledge deemed relevant by the course can usually be discovered from looking at the skills referred to in the assessment format.

It is too early for firm headings for the assessment of community work to emerge but we should at least be beginning to define expectations more precisely and attempting to group the elements of practice in a more logical way.

The introduction of the integrated methods approach into social work training has raised new issues for fieldwork practice and the assessment of it. If it is widely adopted, then courses will be searching for a different kind of experience for their students and this will be reflected in the criteria for assessment. It seems likely that the tendency will be to emphasise knowledge and skill areas common to casework, group and community work while giving a low profile to those areas of knowledge and skill peculiar to each form of intervention. In assessing potential community work practitioners, we need to be looking for competence, not only in common areas of practice but also in those areas which are peculiar to community work.

MOVING TOWARDS A MODEL OF ASSESSMENT

Teaching institutions often request that in long placements there should be one or two interim assessments. This is an improvement on the situation where student and supervisor suddenly realise that there are only another four or five days before an assessment must be done, but it is still not adequate. Assessment has to be a continuous process.[12] The student and supervisor need to use supervision sessions to review progress and discuss the learning opportunities presented by the field situation. The actual written assessment is not particularly important except insofar as it satisfies the requirements of the awarding bodies and compels the supervisor and student to sharpen their judgements.

At least one community work course places the emphasis on self-assessment. Though there are dangers in depending exclusively upon a student's ability to assess his own performance, there should be much more stress than there is on self-assessment. Frequently community workers operate in agencies where they receive neither support nor informed supervision. The worker has to depend upon his own capacity for self-criticism and he is more likely to be capable of this if in his field experience he was encouraged to assess himself.

In America some research – albeit on a small scale – was done to establish whether there was a correlation between certain factors in the performance of social work students. One of the things which emerged was that there is a significant correlation between competence and a high level of self-awareness.[13] In our own field teaching, we have found that – given the opportunity – most students can play a large part in assessing their work and that almost invariably the best students show an ability to be self-critical.

Assuming that supervision sessions have been used in a way which has encouraged the student to engage in a process of continuous self-assessment, then the task of drawing up the final assessment might begin with the student's writing down of his own comments using a format which should have been in his possession from the beginning of the placement. The supervisor might at the same time prepare his own notes or, as we usually do, write notes taking into account the student's own assessment after which there should be a joint session in which they agree – if possible – a document which is acceptable to both of them. If there are minor disagreements which could affect the awarding of a qualification, then the course tutor should be asked to meet with the supervisor and student before the final assessment is completed. In the event of continuing disagreement, then the procedure referred to later would have to be invoked.

Over three years in which more than sixty students have been supervised in our student unit, only on two occasions has it been necessary to involve the course tutor. On another two or three occasions, the course tutor has asked to be involved in a discussion about the final assessment because she has realised that in the light of the student's general performance the assessment on the placement could be of special importance.

It is worth stressing that assessments should begin with a clear statement of the student's assignment. This is particularly important in community work when very often both course tutors and external examiners are very uncertain about the nature of community work.

It is also important because a student's performance can only be evaluated against the opportunities provided by the agency. Already we are in the area of chance. One student is asked to work in an agency and on a project which enables him to use his knowledge and skills to the full. Another is in the kind of agency where he feels uncomfortable and, to make things worse, he is given a task which is fraught with difficulties or a project which – through no fault of the student – peters out half way through his placement. (Often it is a matter of very delicate judgement whether a piece of work comes to nothing because of the failings of the student or because of the nature of the situation.)

ASSESSMENT CRITERIA

A study of assessment criteria drawn up by some twenty social work courses reveals a confused assortment of major headings and detailed guidelines. It is difficult to discern any clear pattern. Some of them obviously attempt to relate the criteria to the current objectives of the course but others have not been modified in the light of curriculum changes and new types of fieldwork. Many courses have, for instance, introduced a community work element but this has not been taken into account in working out fieldwork evaluation headings.

One course in its field teachers' handbook, in arguing against any grading beyond pass or fail, says that this 'is not a flight on the part of the tutors and field teachers from recognition of any objective standards, but, we believe, a recognition that to seek to differentiate between degrees of passing supposes a level of sophistication and control of assessment that we do not yet have'. This is a realistic view. There is no absolute standard. The whole process is relative and must be treated as such by all concerned with it.

It is tempting to offer a format for assessing community work field practice and doubtless this would be appreciated by many course tutors. It would, however, be a mistake. Evaluation guidelines need to be the product of discussions between students, tutors and supervisors which take into account the theoretical orientation of the course, the nature of the placement opportunities and the expectations of all three parties. Presumably one eye must also be kept on the requirements of external examiners.

The most we can do is to indicate some of the general areas which are relevant to field practice in community work. For convenience, we will group under the headings referred to above of knowledge, skills and attitudes. In practice these are interrelated and can be grouped in a variety of ways.

Knowledge of:

> community structures;
> political structures;
> organisational structures;
> resources;
> group processes;
> interpersonal relationships.

Skills in:

> gathering, analysing and using information;
> establishing relationships;
> working with groups;
> interorganisational work;
> communication;
> administration;
> planning strategy;
> organising;
> evaluation.

Attitudes towards:

> agency;
> colleagues;
> other professional workers;
> consumers;
> people with different values;
> those in authority;
> self.

Each of these can be expanded in numerous ways. How we do this and what we look for in the assessment process will be determined by many factors not least of which will be the values of the participants.

CONCLUSION: SAFEGUARDS AND CHECKS IN ASSESSMENT

It is important that safeguards and checks are built into such a fallible process as assessment. Where difficulties are developing in the student – supervisor relationship, it is necessary that a third person should be involved. It is also important that there should be a clearly laid-down arbitration procedure in the event of a major disagreement about the final assessment. This might include a panel which should have on it a representative of the students and a fieldwork supervisor from another agency. Alternatively, both the student and fieldworker should be free to submit their own case to the external examiner. It is unlikely that any such procedure would have to be invoked very often but this makes it no less important that there should be some machinery for dealing with any case which might arise.

REFERENCES

1 Felicity Jackson, 'Fieldwork Supervision', *Case Con*, No. 17, Autumn 1974.

2 Arnold Gurin, *Community Organization Curriculum in Graduate Social Work Education* (Council on Social Work Education, New York, 1970), p. 20.

3 Ibid, p. 21.

4 Social Work Curriculum Study, *The Teaching of Community Work* (Central Council for Education and Training in Social Work, London, 1974), p. 73.

5 G. Williams, 'The Essential Ingredients, and Context of Community Work Supervision', *Supervision in Community Work Placements* (mimeographed report of consultation sponsored by the Joint University Council for Social and Public Administration, 1972), p. 19.

6 Ibid, p. 16.

7 B. Holmes, R. Bryant and D. Houston, 'Student Unit in Community Work: An 'Experimental Approach', *Social Work Today*, vol. 4, No. 10 (1973).

8 Philip Evens, 'Community Work Supervision and the Casework model', *Community Work – Theory and Practice* (Alistair Shornach Ltd., Oxford, 1974), p. 132f.

9 Peter Baldock, 'Community Work Experience in Social Work Training', in Jones and Mayo (eds), *Community Work One* (Routledge & Kegan Paul, 1974), pp. 233 and 238.

10 Felicity Jackson, op. cit.

11 Priscilla Young, *The Student and Supervision in Social Work Education* (Routledge & Kegan Paul, 1967), p. 105.

12 Social Work Curriculum Study, *The Teaching of Community Work* (Central Council for Education and Training in Social Work, London, 1974), p. 64.

13 'Trends in Fieldwork Instruction', reprinted from *Social Casework* (Family Service Association, America).

FURTHER READING

Brown, Clements S. and Gloyne, E. R., *The Field Training of Social Workers* (George Allen & Unwin, 1966).

Gurin, Arnold, *Community Organization Curriculum in Graduate Social Work Education* (Council on Social Work Education, New York, 1970).

Pettes, Dorothy E., *Supervision in Social Work* (George Allen & Unwin, 1967).

Towle, Charlotte, *The Learner in Education for the Professions As seen in Education for Social Work* (University of Chicago Press, 1954).

Young, Priscilla, *The Student and Supervision in Social Work Education* (Routledge & Kegan Paul, 1967).

Social Work Curriculum Study, *The Teaching of Community Work* (Central Council for Education and Training in Social Work, 1974).

Chapter 12

INTRAROLE CONFLICT AND A CASEWORK–COMMUNITY WORK COMPOSITE ROLE

Jalna Hanmer

This chapter comments on the observations of students on their experiences in moving to and from casework and community work method placements on one social work course over the past two years.

The course was for postgraduates, for one academic year, with two consecutive placements of three days a week. The course was organised around methods of social work. Placements were designated casework, group work or community work and each student was concurrently a member of a similarly designated methods class when in the school. Two placements enabled some students to choose to gain experience in two methods. All students had prior work experience, occasionally in more than one method, or in community work only; most had specialised in casework.

Exposure to a new method had several results. While students reacted differently to the experience of occupying and changing to and from the roles of caseworker and community worker, most students experienced considerable anxiety in their efforts to find out what was expected of them. Yet on occasion a student could feel immediately at home, confirming a prior sense that 'this is for me', thus enabling the student to define the other more familiar method as inappropriate for him/her. Another response was more ambivalent: while experiencing a placement in the familiar method as a slot easier to fill, or more 'normal', a student could still feel like a fish out of water when moving from the unfamiliar method back to the familiar one.

The aim of this chapter is to explore, in a preliminary way, the student's subjective comprehension of the roles of caseworker and community worker.[1] The comments of students ranged from the role activity itself to their expectations for the role behaviour of staff and fieldwork supervisors of the course and to the theoretical perspectives associated with casework and community work.

INTRAROLE CONFLICT

The phenomenon of feeling like a casework student in a community work placement and, alternatively, of feeling like a community work student in a casework placement is a subjective experience of intrarole conflict.[2] Intrarole conflict arises when there are contradictory expectations for the same role held by one or more groups of relevant others, for example caseworkers and community workers for the role of social worker.[3] To the extent that students saw the role of social worker as embracing both the activities of caseworkers and community workers the problem of the integration of the two was sharply posed.

The potential for intrarole conflict is maximised when helping individuals in a community-work setting or when helping a category of clients in a casework placement. The conflict can be so extreme that the inappropriate activity is either avoided or reclassified into the other if it occurs. Thus students on a community work placement may almost furtively help an individual with a particular problem, for instance gas board arrears. In casework placements the situation at its most extreme can be worse as the constraint may not operate on the level of action but on that of thought, so that social explanations and potential solutions are not even offered for discussion for fear of censure. On our course the problem of intrarole conflict for students was lessened somewhat as the roles of caseworker and community worker were enacted successively during a given time period. Yet the fact that these two roles were successive ultimately made their integration more difficult.

Some students may claim to experience the process of taking on the roles of caseworker and community worker as one of taking on the outer facade provided by the other's expectations: for example, 'I think it is much more important how people see you rather than how you feel in these situations'; and 'I can only be the same person, the other party projected a different image on to me'. This mechanistic conception of role process, however, does not seem to do justice to the experience of students as individual variation indicates that the roles of caseworker and community worker are not fixed entities into which the individual slots, but arise out of reciprocal interaction. The process, to use Turner's phrase, is one of role making not role taking, and is a process based on discovering and creating consistent wholes out of behaviour.[4] Roles conceived of in this way are comprehensive alternative ways of dealing with a given other role, and role making consists of the successful anticipation of behaviour of relevant others within a range necessary for enactment of one's own role. Thus students do not simply learn detailed prescriptions for behaviour, but, within a general framework, work out appropriate role behaviour.

The initial uncertainty of students when first in a community work placement may focus on being deprived of the authority implicit in the title 'social worker for X social services department' or in no longer having statutory duties. For some students the worker's authority in relation to clients seemed to stem from a different source, or at least to be less agency-, statute-, and custom-based. Alternatively, students in a casework situation for the first time did feel the authority implicit in their new role particularly burdensome.

The issue of authority can be raised in many ways. It can be the focus for sudden knowledge of what it means to be in a different role. One student when visiting a woman about a tenants' association matter found himself in the familiar one-to-one position. Suddenly he remembered that she had a child in the care of the local authority and thought how inappropriate, while in the community work role, it would be to ask her about her income or sexual life – both suitable topics if he were her local authority caseworker. This student was acutely aware that to ask such questions would be to step out of role so seriously as to jeopardise his credibility as an adequate community worker and, he believed, at the very least would result in his being thrown out of her flat. The source and exercise of authority is one important variable, and, to the extent that students interpret the casework role as that of a good parent, they may contrast the community work role as that of a good sibling.[5]

The same dichotomy may be applied to the student–supervisor relationship: 'I was used to an authoritarian approach (as a hospital social worker) and found a non-directive approach from my community work supervisor confusing'; and 'as a community work student you are left to find your own feet – given a free hand – and I was not used to that!' Also, students believed that the acquisition of the community work and casework roles meant different styles of learning. They saw the community work role as involving more stress – 'very uncomfortable while you are doing it but there is no other way' – and felt that 'a certain amount of the process just has to happen – of setting to a situation and picking it up'. Yet this point of view was also echoed by students in a statutory casework agency for the first time, particularly by those with only a community work background. Thus it may be possible that a major factor in the interpretation of the learning process is whether or not one is an absolute beginner.

As has been widely noted, one basic difference between casework and community work is between a psychological (or micro-) or a sociological (or macro-) orientation to social facts.[6] Social workers can spontaneously shift from one perspective to the other as this student's example illustrates: 'In the local authority setting in which I worked (before coming on the course) I was encouraged to view these mothers (unmarried and on supplementary benefit) as having personality problems of very different types and not encouraged to look at their common difficulties in surviving on a low income in a generally unaccepting environment.' Thus her initial view of why a young, black, mother did not pay her rent was because 'she did not trust authority figures in general' and building relationships of trust with her was seen as a way of overcoming her resistance. After a few months of visiting, 'I thought she was beginning to accept that not all figures of authority were bad and that her self-esteem was much higher than when I first knew her'; yet her rent arrears were increasing. The point of transition to a new analysis came when, with her encouragement, the client found the best job she could along with a place at a nursery for her one-year-old son. Yet 'going out to work did help not J. pay her rent as there was no increase in income. She occupied a position in society, as I now saw it, where whatever she did her income would not substantially rise.' Thus the analytic focus sifted from personality difficulties to factors associated with colour, sex and social class.

An awareness of this kind of shift in perception may also occur when students change their placement. For instance, one student, previously employed as a caseworker, described her initial reaction to a casework placement after having spent six months, three days a week, in community work thus: 'I noticed that nearly all clients were either black or else they were shrivelled, humble and elderly.' Everyday events in agency management were used to assess client status: 'I noted that the sixteen social workers, clerks and typists occupied four large rooms while the clients were interviewed either on the landing or in a tiny old fashioned kitchen . . . Social workers walked briskly to and fro, often carrying cups of coffee which were never offered to the clients.' Court work was seen with new eyes: 'I found it impossible to see the courts in any other terms than as the middle classes sitting in judgement on the poor', as was school phobia: 'In the courts it was invariably seen as the child's fault or the parent's fault, never that of the school.'

While her initial reaction was to think of social workers sharing the coffee and a room in order to free one for interviewing, the student recorded a quick return to becoming accustomed to the 'sight of a mute black person on the landing patiently waiting to be seen'. Further, when allocated cases that were neither particularly poor nor suffering from bad housing conditions she became convinced that the majority presented problems that could only be solved by careful listening and analysis with a genuine effort to understand their history and present situation. She reported that sharpened perceptions of the internal patterns of people's lives led on occasion to a real vision of their difficulties, a clear understanding of the connection between their past and present: 'It gave me a feeling of elation to see these connections, whether I shared these intuitions with my clients or kept them to myself.' Thus this student moved from a micro- to a macro- and back to a micro-orientation to clients.

Developing and applying both a psychological and sociological focus at one and the same time to the same phenomena seems to be akin to being ambidextrous, and is probably just as rare.[7] Why this is so needs examination. Those who argue that the theoretical underpinning for casework and community work is the same (i.e. the social sciences) and thus that casework and community work are of the same genre, conveniently overlook the fact that the exact nature of the interrelationship between the disciplines that make up the social sciences remains obscure.[8] While there may be a level of generality on which all is complementary, more specific explanations of human conduct can be presented as alternatives; the relationship between disciplines and their theories can be as conflictual as that between the various methods of social work intervention.

A lower level of abstraction simply repeats the same pattern so that the perspective of complementarity applied to the social work task (for instance, Evens's description of the continuum as ranging from preventing breakdown to promoting welfare with an overlap somewhere in the middle) suffers from the same covert conflict.[9] Thus the relevant theories, with their lack of integration, may make it difficult for the individual to use simultaneously the various micro- and macro-theoretical perspectives as a basis for action.

While it may be a truism that both psychological and sociological perspectives are equally valid and needed at one and same time, this does not obviate the intrarole conflict that arises on attempting to put these perspectives into practice. As we all know there is a crucial difference between them: one facilitates an analysis of personal inadequacy while the other enables a focus to be made on societal inadequacy. In practice a number of outcomes are possible; to accomplish improvement in the individual or social area may or may not result in improvement in both and, further, improvement may be made more unlikely by 'cooling out' individuals. Thus practice, too, makes its own contribution to intrarole conflict.

As we all know, community work students on a social work course can be the most dissatisfied; as Sarbin explains, the results of cognitive strain associated with role conflict are 'low job satisfaction, little confidence in the organisation and high tension related to the job'.[10]

SOLUTIONS TO INTRAROLE CONFLICT

Students varied in their interest in attempting, and success in achieving, a personally satisfactory integration of casework and community work both at the conceptual and practice skill level. The connections between theory and practice, casework and community work are fourfold (Figure 12.1).

Students may claim that academic methods teaching is of little relevance to the practice of either method and/or be unable to see any links between them. Students may conclude that they have been learning what was demanded in their particular practical situation only, and, while social work educators may console themselves with the thought that it is a slow and individual digestive process to be completed long after the student leaves the course, the cry that 'nothing seems to hang together' obviously raises issues about the course itself as well as the nature of the two roles.

By offering students disparate theoretical and practical experiences intrarole conflict is increased. One solution open to the student is to ignore the problem of consistency by compartmentalising knowledge and experience. Compartmentalising can be both an inner psychological and an outer behavioural response. One well-known way of coping is to idealise community work and reject casework, a response more likely to succeed if supported by the student culture on the course.

The role of the fieldworker supervisor, as well as that of course staff, is also important in increasing or decreasing the ease of compartmentalising on the part of students. Adverse comments by casework supervisors about community work and vice versa, or the occasional refusal by caseworker agencies to take students who have had community work placements, for instance, all help to create a course climate that encourages compartmentalising and thus makes integration that much more difficult. Further, to the student it may feel like a lack of concern: 'How can a course have casework supervisors who do not understand the difficulties that students on community work placements are having? How can a social worker be like that?' Alternatively, the view of some community supervisors that community work is not social work, without offering any alternative explanation of what it then is, increases role conflict: 'I was not sure what was positively expected of me, only that I must not behave like a caseworker, or a leader, or a full-time member of any of the groups I attended, nor should I take on any long term commitments.'

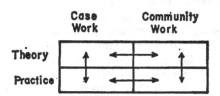

Figure 12.1

An alternative way of dealing with role conflict is to merge conflicting roles into a single new compromise role. The single role may result from a merger process, each role absorbing the other, or from the development and recognition of a third role which is specifically the pattern viewed as consistent when both roles might be applicable. The recent theoretical contributions using a social systems approach are an important attempt to develop a conceptual basis for a composite role that includes casework, group work and community work.[11]

Student suggestions on how to improve the integration of casework and community work roles focused on reducing the ease with which the individual can compartmentalise experiences. On the level of practice students suggested mixed method placements, or two contrasting placements in the same area – 'we can then look at the area from two angles' – or a more gradual introduction through a mixed method placement followed by an unstructured community work one.

In practice, partial integration was more likely, and given favourable experiences students could make a connection between theory and practice on the level of values:[12] 'There is a similarity between the non-directive method in community work and acceptance and refusal to judge people in casework. I have been fortunate in having both casework and community work supervisors who have tried diligently to put these principles into practice.' Another technique was for students to redefine their beliefs about casework, or community work, so that the roles became more compatible. Community work placements then could be seen as valuable for training caseworkers: 'Having done some community work I will approach casework in an entirely different way.'

While students seemed to strive after role synthesis, not all experience of it was felt as positive. Students tended to see the community worker as a different kind of person – one with a more overt political outlook – and community work as a means of large-scale change. The conclusion that 'community work isn't going to change a deprived state and I think that is the kind of illusion I was under when I started out', even if a realistic assessment, is depressing for the individual.

The argument, however, is not that the consequence of the similarity between casework and community work is that neither can result in positive change, but rather that the process of social work intervention between work with the individual and collectivity is experienced as discontinuous. Work with the community, but apparently not with the individual, is seen as an essentially political process in which concepts of power, interest and conflict are necessarily present. It would seem, however, that these factors are subliminal, rather than absent, in casework.

It is tempting to apply Pearson's argument on knowledge about power as the repressed content of social work practice to the experience of students.[13] As Pearson explains the exercise of power in the client-worker relationship is never made explicit except in a truncated form as 'authority'. By making explicit the routine grounds of decision making in welfare bureaucracies, repressed knowledge surfaces, as this action de-routinises the professional culture of social work with its built-in conception of the world. What Pearson describes as the interpenetrations of professionalism, power, interest, conflict, morality and economy with social work, then begin to be exposed. Thus community work potentially becomes an Achilles' heel, and not just for the profession but for the individual. Looked at in this way it is not surprising that frequently the subjective experience of intrarole conflict of students is focused around the issue of authority.

Students undertaking placements in more than one social work method carry out conscious knowledge of the intrarole conflict involved. As a first step towards a greater understanding and possibly, ultimately, a resolution of it, those of us in social work education, both caseworkers and community workers, need to make this knowledge our own. The task, however, is made more difficult by the degree to which compartmentalising is used as a solution to role conflict by social work teachers and fieldwork supervisors.

Yet more is needed than goodwill. A greater use of mixed methods in the field is encouraging as are experiment and change within courses. On our own course, for instance, students, supervisors and tutors are becoming involved in an experimental group on teaching methods with special reference to the relationship between casework, group work and community work.

CONCLUSION

In this chapter an attempt has been made to look at the experience of students in terms of role theory. To accept explicitly that the process of learning about casework and community work is one of role acquisition with inherent intrarole conflict is to recognise structural factors clearly and it may be one way of helping students, supervisors and tutors to look again at student experiences. We need to examine more closely how roles are negotiated and what happens to the knowledge students have of power, interest and conflict as they move from working with individuals to the collectivity.

NOTES AND REFERENCES

1 As the aim is to cast light on intrarole conflict and not the differences between the reactions of students, individual factors such as students' previous employment, general life experiences and personality are not discussed.

2 T. R. Sarbin and V. L. Allen, 'Role Theory', in G. Lindzey and E. Aronson (eds), *Handbook of Social Psychology* (Addison-Wesley, 1969) 2nd edn, vol. 1, p. 540.

3 While for the purposes of social work education social work is conceived as a composite role including specific role activity called case-, group and community work, as we all know within the profession social work is defined both as casework only and more broadly to include both group and community work. While some social workers may exhibit unflagging consistency in one or the other interpretation, inconsistency is probably nearer the norm, which both illustrates the complexity and complicates our understanding of the issues involved.

4 R. H. Turner, 'Role-Taking: Process versus Conformity', in A. M. Rose (ed.), *Human Behaviour and Social Processes* (London, Routledge & Kegan Paul, 1962), pp. 20–40.

5 Community literature certainly lends support to this type of thinking. Community work polemic is firmly egalitarian in tone, while writings on casework explicitly refer to good parenting as an aspect of the role. For example, M. Brown, 'A Review of Casework Methods', in E. Younghusband (ed.), *New Developments in Casework* (George Allen & Unwin, 1966), pp. 11–38.

6 For example, P. Evens, *Community Work Theory and Practice* (Oxford, Alistair Shornach Ltd, 1974), p. 50.

7 There is another sense in which ambidexterity can be used as a simile. Casework can be equated with introversion. 'You have to delve into yourself to find out what casework is about'; while community work is equated with extroversion: 'For a community worker everything depends on your powers of observation' and 'You are trying to achieve particular tasks and somehow the relationship bit goes along by default'. But even if it is a question of projecting mutually exclusive categories on to casework and community work, they are not entirely inappropriate and inaccurate.

8 M. Rein, 'The Cross-roads for Social Work', *Social Work*, vol. 27, No. 4, 1970, p. 19, describes the implications of this: 'Although we have theories about society and theories about individuals, we have few theories to link both together. Thus no matter how much the dichotomy offends common sense we continue to teach students each body of literature unrelated to the other.'

9 P. Evens, op. cit.

10 Sarbin and Allen, op. cit., p. 543.

11 A. Pincus and A. Minahan, *Social Work Practice: Model and Method* (Illinois, Peacock Publ., 1973).
   H. Goldstein, *Social Work Practice: A Unitary Approach* (South Carolina, University of South Carolina, 1973).

12 Role activities of caseworkers can be described in similar terms to those used for community workers. For example see Florence Hollis, 'The Psychosocial approach to the Practice of Casework' in R. W. Roberts and R. H. Nee (eds), *Theories of Social Casework* (University of Chicago Press, 1970), p. 63. When this happens, however, the argument about role differences switches from the type of activity undertaken by the worker to the number of clients dealt with at any one time, one only or a group.

13 G. Pearson, 'The Politics of Uncertainty: a study in the socialisation of the social worker', in H. Jones (ed.), *Towards a New Social Work* (Routledge & Kegan Paul, 1975), pp. 45–68.

POSTWORD

There is a persistent theme which runs through many of the chapters in this book. It calls on community workers to reflect upon their work and to develop a critical consciousness and appraisal of:

the material world, and the economic and social arrangements that perpetuate powerlessness and poverty;
theories and knowledge about that world;
the potential and the limitations of community work as an intervention in situations of economic and social deprivation;
the mechanisms (e.g. supervision, training courses) through which intervention is developed and strengthened.

It is one of our basic assumptions as trainers that action without reflection in community work can harm the interests of community groups. Trainers and practitioners have a responsibility to improve both their work and their ability to think about that work. We believe with one contributor to this book that 'the fusing of theory and practice, where understanding the work and changing it are part of the same process, should be a major objective of community work itself.'

INDEX

Agencies, relationship with community workers 24–8, 29, 33, 42, 46, 48, 49–50, 125, 171
Algorithms 126
Assessment of students 155, 158, 168–76
Association of Community Workers 13, 56, 58

Body language, *see* Groups: Communication systems

Casework and community work 150, 178–85
Central Council for Education and Training in Social Work 13
Citizens' Rights Office 38
Collaborative strategy 127–8
Collective behaviour, *see* Groups: Large groups
Community Action 13
Community and Youth Service Association 58, 59
Community Development Information Group, Liverpool 56
Community Development Projects 13, 43
Community groups (*see also* Groups): Goals 82, 85, 119; Policy criteria 123–4; Strategies 119, 125–9
Community integration 127–8
Community work: Administration 34–5; As a recognised field 30, 59; Class approach to research 114–15; Compared to case work 178–85; Consultancy process 51–3; Contribution of social sciences 69–79; Controversial issues 13–15, 67; Courses 137; Differing expectations 40, 42; Empiricism in research 113–14, 115; Fieldwork teaching 149–50, 151–66; Goals 26, 45–6, 50–1; Growth of interest 13; Management studies 118–33; Methodology 129–32; Models of community problems 75–7; Planning 45–6, 119; Practice framework 77–8, 79; Priori-

ties 136; 'Professionalisation' 13–15, 33, 56, 68; Project analysis 105; Research methods 104–16; Simulation 130–32, 144, 151; Strategies 125–29; Teaching, *see* Community workers: students; Theory and practice 70–1, 77–8, 138, 143
Community workers: As agents of social change 14, 16, 33, 41–2, 49, 51; Authority 27–8; Consultants 21, 23, 24, 31, 41, 43–55; Data: Recording 112, 113, 114, 115; Sources 109–10, 113; Discussion opportunities 23, 24–5, 26, 30, 31–2, 35, 160; Field practice 16, 34, 35; Grant applications 105; Groups 21, 22, 31–2, 56–63; Organisation 56; Training function 58–9, 62; In-service training 21, 23, 30–1, 60–2; Interviewing 111–12; Investigation techniques 112–13; Knowledge and skills 13, 15, 16, 21, 24, 32, 36–8, 46–8, 129–30, 136–45, 154–5, 172–3; Observation in research 108–9, 164; Personal characteristics 36, 41, 47–8, 144; Personal goals 144–5; Project analysis 105; Relationship with agencies, *see* Agencies; Research approach 105–7; Resources 35, 38; Roles 28, 37, 94, 125–9, 179–85; Skills, *see* Community workers: Knowledge and skills; Stress 25, 29, 33, 38–9, 56, 180; Students 149–50, 151–85; Assessment 155, 158, 168–76; Course expectations 170–2; Fieldwork 149–50, 152–66, 169; Learning and experience 136–45; Learning situations 159–65; Placement 155–9; Supervision 21, 23, 24, 26–7, 28–30, 33–42, 60–2, 145, 152–3, 159–60, 165, 170, 174, 183; Surveys 110–13; Training: Direct experience model 136–45; Opportunities 15, 16, 21, 30–1, 33, 46–8, 60–3; Understanding 140–1, 143
Consultants, *see* Community workers
Co-ordinative strategy 127

Printed in the United States
by Baker & Taylor Publisher Services